Newcastle

Short Story Award

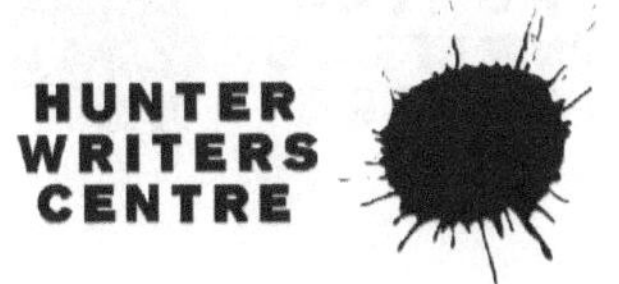

First published in Australia in 2018 by Hunter Writers Centre
www.hunterwriterscentre.org

Newcastle Short Story Award Anthology 2018
ISBN: 978-0-9954409-3-7

Cover photograph by Shane Williams
https://strikingnewcastle.com.au

Published by Hunter Writers Centre Inc. 2018

Hunter Writers Centre Newcastle NSW 2300
info@hunterwriterscentre.orghunterwriterscentre.org

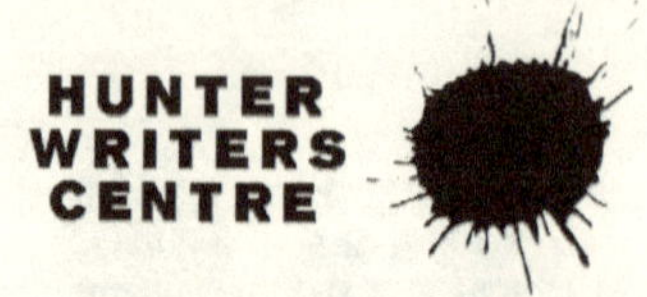

Table of Contents

Judges' Foreword

There are two kinds of people in the world; those who read short stories, and those who should read short stories.

If you have bought this book, the odds are that you are in the first group, and need no further persuasion as to the merits of reading short fiction; you will perhaps find yourself nodding as you read this foreword. But if by some chance you are in the second group, one of those people who say, "I just can't get into short stories; I prefer novels" then grant us the opportunity to change your mind in the next five hundred words.

A short story isn't a novel, and neither is it inferior to a novel. This may seem self-evident, but it is still worth pointing out, as sometimes short fiction is thought of as the novel's poorer cousin (and certainly it can feel that way when trying to get a short story collection published). There remain some who see the short story as little more than a set of literary training wheels, to be used only long enough for the fledgling writer to gain enough confidence so that they can get on with the real business of writing, that is, writing a novel.

But the truth is that writing a short story is nothing like writing with a set of training wheels; to strain the analogy, it is more like riding a unicycle, upon which the writer is balanced, juggling six balls in the air, and another on their nose. A novelist has hundreds of pages to create their characters, establish their setting, crank the plot into motion. A short story writer has only a few thousand words. A novelist can afford the occasional cliché, or a flat patch which the reader skims over quickly in the hope the book gets good again soon. A short story writer has no such luxury. Everything has to work, and in the best short stories, everything does work, so well that the reader is unaware of the skill required. And this is the magic of the short story; it creates a world, peoples it with characters and tells a story that effortlessly carries the reader along from beginning to end. A good short story provides a jolt of experience, a glimpse into another life that lingers like an afterimage, and one of the pleasures of reading an anthology of stories such as this one is encountering a wide variety of images, styles, characters, plots and worlds. It was certainly one of the pleasures of selecting the stories that went into this anthology.

Now in its third consecutive year, the Newcastle Short Story Award received hundreds of entries from all over the country. It was an enormous task to read such a huge number and one that was stimulating, surprising, and sometimes exhausting. With such a large number of entries, it is perhaps no surprise that common themes should emerge which were explored by a number of writers in different ways. Childhood, for example, was a setting for dozens of stories, and while many of these were authentically imagined, they could often read more like reminiscences than a short story with a beginning, middle and end. A great number of stories began with the protagonist waking up; this did not mean that the story was bad, but perhaps indicates that this opening gambit has become some- thing of a default, and more thought is needed to capture the reader's attention. Perhaps the most common theme that emerged was that of family, how they hurt, and sometimes how they heal.

Over several weeks the judges read each story separately, before coming up with two separate longlists of about sixty stories each, with some overlap in their choices. After some discussion, this longlist was slowly whittled down to the 32 stories that appear in this anthology. There was a short break to let the stories settle, and then the shortlisted stories were read once again, and the winning entries chosen. There was little disagreement between the judges at the this stage; while there were several strong contenders, both judges agreed that Shaynah Andrews wonderfully tender 'Not For Me to Understand' was a clear winner. This is not to take anything away from Cassie Hamer's heart-breaking 'Sculptures by the Sea' in second place, or Jean Flynn's astute 'Suffering is Universal' in third, both of which are fine stories, and could well have won in a different year.

Well, it appears we have reached the end of the foreword. If you insist on remaining in the camp of those who claim they don't particularly enjoy short stories, then I just happen to have the perfect book that I guarantee will change your mind.

Read on.

Ryan O'Neill and Isabelle Li

Awards

First Prize *donated by the University of Newcastle*
Not For Me To Understand - *Shaynah Andrews, NSW*

Second Prize *donated by The Newcastle Law Society*
Sculptures By The Sea - *Cassie Hamer, NSW*

Third Prize *donated by Westfield Kotara*
Suffering Is Universal - *Jean Flynn, Vic*

Highly Commended *donated by Foghorn Brewhouse*
Red Belly - *Jane O'Sullivan, NSW*

Highly Commended *donated by Maclean's Booksellers*
Excess Baggage - *Tanya Vavilova, NSW*

Commended *donated by Elliot Watson Financial Planning*
Postcard - *Wayne Strudwick, ACT*

Commended *donated by Dymocks*
Dachshunds on antidepressants - *M.J. Reidy, NSW*

Local Awards: *Stephanie Holm Edyn Carter Rhona Hammond Shaynah Andrews*

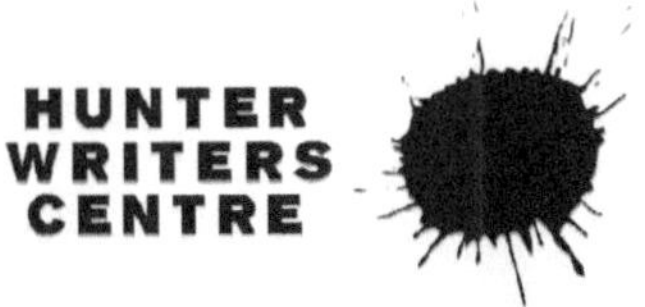

Newcastle Short Story Award Sponsors

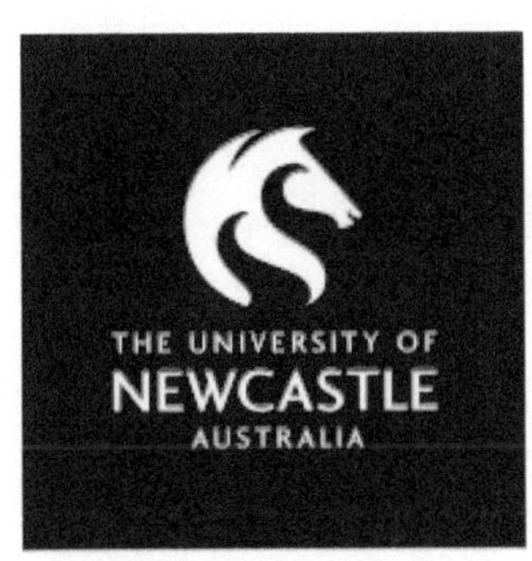

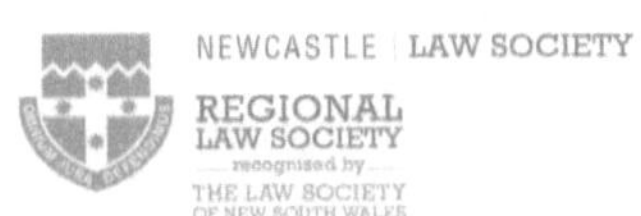

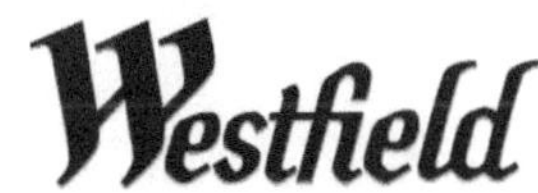

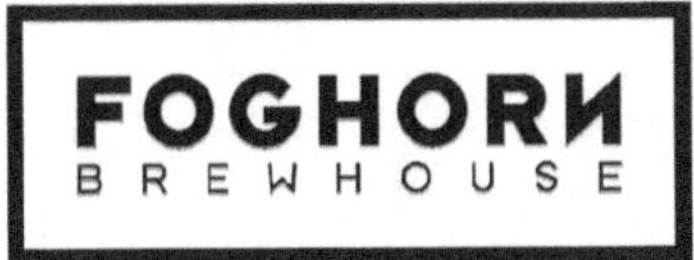

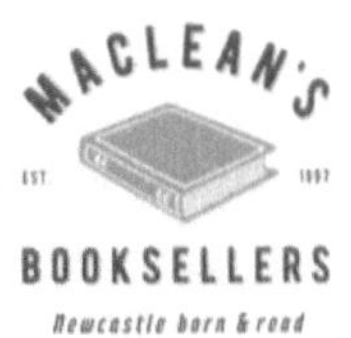

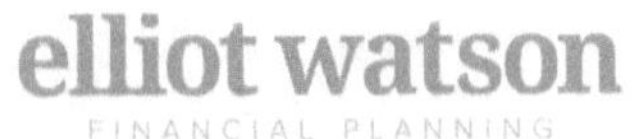

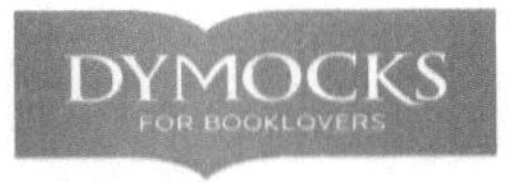

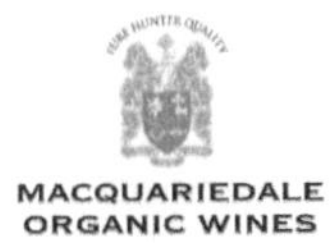

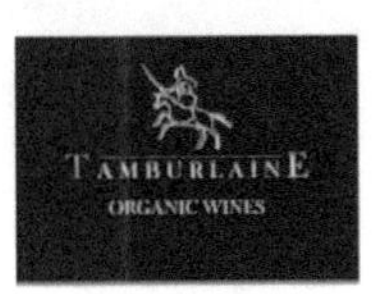

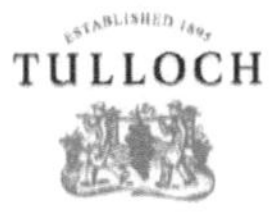

Not for Me to Understand

Shaynah Andrews

First Prize

Dad nicks me with the clippers when he shaves my head. Hot ash from his cigarette brushes my ear before it hits the ground. I run my hand over, after, and it feels like the dog's coat after a bath. Rough and soft at the same time. My fingers find blood.

My brother, Jacob, laughs at the mound of curls at my toes. 'Lil, you look like a little boy!'

Dad growls at him. 'It's what my Mum did when I had nits as a kid. Sorry, possum,' he says.

'I don't think our Mum would have done this, Dad,' I say.

'Well, is she here to ask?' He has a face like people get before they cry.

I put my arms around his neck. 'Don't worry, Dad. It's school holidays. It'll grow back.'

On Tuesdays we get works burgers from the fish and chip shop. Jacob manages to eat two even though he's skinny as a rake. Dad lets Jacob have a VB but I can tell he only pretends to like it from the way his eyes wrinkle up when he takes a sip. We watch M*A*S*H* with Dad. I like Radar the best. Dad reminds me of Hawkeye because he's always mucking around. And he always has different girlfriends over but there are no girlfriends invited to hamburger Tuesdays.

There is still light out 'til late, so, after M*A*S*H I help Dad hang all the sheets out on the clothesline. Jacob kicks around a football with our cattle dog Ellie. The breeze feels nice against my naked head.

We ride our pushies to the beach carpark, Jacob in front. Ellie follows us but she is old and slow, so we have to circle back to her every so often just to make sure she doesn't get left behind on the road.

There's a small mystery to do with our faces. Jacob and I look almost exactly the same as each other: green eyes, freckles, the same shape to our features except his nose and ears are a little bigger. But everybody says I look just like my Mum did and Jacob looks just like Dad. This feels like a trick to me. I wonder if now my hair is short like a boy people will stop saying that I look like Mum. I don't ask Jacob, who gets angry now whenever anybody talks about her.

Jacob is fifteen but he still lets me ride with him so long as I keep to myself. I have loads of practice making myself small, almost invisible. Jacob's tyres screech as he brakes hard at the bottom of the carpark. He chucks a move where his front wheel stops sharp and the back wheel goes up in the air like he is a cowboy on the saddle of a bucking horse. Jacob lands and waves over one of his friends who is waiting for him.

'Who's this?' Danny asks. He is holding a skateboard under his arm. His pants sit so low on his hip bones that I can see the way his muscles form a V leading down into his underwear. I look away.

'It's Lil, you dickhead,' Jacob says.

'Oh, shiiit. Where's your hair gone, little sis'?' Danny reaches out and rubs his hand against my head. It hurts a little where the clippers cut me. 'You look like a hard nut now.'

Jacob's girlfriend Anna works at the kiosk attached to the surf club. We chain up our bikes outside and sit on the white plastic seats that look out at the waves. Anna has thick brown hair almost to her waist. The afternoon light paints it in a hundred different colours. She gives us free icy poles when her manager isn't around. She knows my favourite is lemonade. I watch her as she leans over the steel countertop to talk to Jacob. Her big smile is white and kind. I've heard Jacob talk about her new boobs to his friends and I feel shameful sneaking glances at them in her polo top. I look down at my bony chest and cannot imagine that it will ever look the way Anna's does.

'Lil! You look like Deb from Empire Records,' Anna says, handing me a lemonade icy pole. 'I love it. Makes your eyes stand out.'

I feel blood rush to my face.

'I told her she looks like a boy,' Jacob says, touching Anna's collar across the counter.

Anna purses her lips. 'Well, girls can look any way they want to, so get used to it, baby.'

Danny pipes up. 'I reckon she looks cool.'

I get a feeling that both boys feel a certain way about Anna but I say nothing to Jacob.

There is a dry heat in the air. The sweet liquid from the icy poles runs down our forearms. We trace it with our tongues. Ellie licks at the syrup gliding down my leg. Gulls taunt her with their ugly sounds.

Anna is closing up the kiosk when Jacob warns us not to follow them. Jacob takes Anna's hand and they set off along the beach. Jacob turns to give Danny a look; a wild look that is not for me to understand. The couple disappears around a bend. It feels like they are gone for a very long time. Danny is still next to me, looking annoyed, when the sun is low over the dunes. Ellie can't see too good in the dark, so I know we'll have to get outta there soon.

'What do you think they're doing?' Danny asks me. 'I dunno,' I say. 'Talkin'. Kissin'.'

'Ha. They've gone off to the sand dunes for a root. He's been planning it.'

'Okay,' I say, not knowing what he means by this exactly but knowing enough to feel squirmy in my seat. I don't want to hang around with Danny. 'I have to get home before dark. Will ya let Jacob know?'

'Righto, little sis.'

There is lead in my belly as I watch Danny clenching and unclenching his fists, breathing loudly like a beast. I can see that he is mad at my brother for having the thing he wants for himself.

I wake in the night to murmurs in the kitchen. Jacob is home and Dad is awake. It sounds like Jacob is sobbing. I have never heard his voice come out so strained; whiny like a scared dog. I can't make out much of their conversation through the walls but I hear Jacob say something like now she's saying she didn't want it, we had a huge fight and dad is saying slow down and you need to tell me exactly what happened. I don't sleep. Instead, I pick at the paint on my bedroom wall that is cracked and curling at the edges. I pick at it until it sticks me under my nails and there is blood.

Jacob has a cut on his lip. I touch my own lip in the place his is bruised and swollen, just to check. Nobody tells me a thing but Jacob packs a backpack and leaves for Gloucester. Our uncle has a farm up there where we go camping every Christmas holidays and spend our days tubing down the river and chasing dogs and letting off New Year's crackers under the stars.

'Is he going to live there from now on?' I ask.

Dad presses the bottoms of his palms to his forehead, impa- tient with my question. 'Lil, I don't know what's gonna happen, OK? It's better this than sending him to some—,' He doesn't finish his sentence. He waves his hands around and shakes his head.

I can feel hot tears coming on and I try my best to stop them. 'Why won't you tell me anything?'

'Because you're too bloody young to know about this kind of shit, possum. I wish you never had to know.' He looks the way Hawkeye does when all the jokes are over.

Dad's new girlfriend, Linda, comes to hamburger Tuesdays now. She orders a veggie patty instead of meat and makes fun of Dad by patting his belly where it is a little soft at the bottom. The first time she comes she rubs my shaved head. I am tired of people touching me. Jacob wouldn't have let Linda come to hamburger Tuesdays.

'Hey Lily, nothing compares to you!' she says, laughing.

Dad laughs too but I don't get the joke. I leave half of my burger and it bleeds through the paper bag.

Later, I hear them talk in low voices from the kitchen. Linda says Maybe she went along with it at first but changed her mind after. Dad says I've known her for years. She's not that sort of girl. Maybe it's all my fault for not talking enough about these things with him.

I can't keep still. I ring the number on the fridge for my uncle's farm house but I get the answering machine. I wonder if Jacob is feeling sorry for himself. He's probably baling hay in the heat all day but I still imagine he's floating on a tube down the river without me, sleeping under the enormous sky, telling his secrets to the dogs.

My blood feels too hot. I want to beat my fists against Dad for treating me like a kid. I smash a cup on the kitchen tiles, half on purpose. There are little bits of glass all around me. Dad and Linda rush into the room.

'I'm sorry, it was an accident,' I say. 'It's OK, possum,' says Dad.

I want him to yell and scream at me but he is gentle.

'I'll clean this up darlin', just get away from all the glass. Careful now.'

Dad and Linda hover over plastic dustpans. I walk out the front door and ride my pushie to the beach with Ellie behind me.

Anna is working the kiosk. She looks distracted, resting her elbows on the countertop and gazing out at the ocean.

'Hey,' I say. 'Are you OK?'

Her body jolts like she gets an electric shock.

'Sorry, Lil. I'm somewhere else today,' she says. 'Want a rainbow Billabong or something?' Her smile doesn't go all the way to her eyes. I scan her for bruises but her hurt is not something I can see like that.

I ask for chocolate. Rainbow is for kids.

Anna asks me if I have heard from Jacob. I tell her not since he left and I tell her that I am lost like I was when Mum died and everybody tried to keep me safe from it all.

She doesn't look at me when she says 'I thought your brother was different but they're all the fucking same. Don't forget that, Lil. Boys are all the same. Think they're entitled to every damn thing.'

I touch her arm but my fingers are sticky with chocolate. 'Sorry,' I say.

She looks at me with pain in her eyes. She studies my face very hard. 'God, you look like him,' she says. It sounds thick in her throat.

I say goodbye to Anna and take Ellie down to the sand to throw a stick around. I think about the times that people couldn't look me in the eye because I reminded them of someone else. For a long time after Mum died Dad would look at me and cry. So, for ages he just stopped looking.

My eyes keep going back to Anna. I watch her refill the plastic straws and napkins on the countertop. Her eyes are heavy. There is no sunlight in her hair. The grey surf churns. Anna keeps trying too hard not to look. I feel something, like the tension before a storm. Hot, heavy air. I run my hand over my hair and it has a new texture, like it's grown some already. I feel a hundred kinds of longing.

Sculptures by the Sea

Cassie Hamer

Second Prize

Stan wanted to walk all the way from Bondi Junction train station to the beach but Carmel wouldn't hear of it.

Her arthritic knees, after all.

So, here they are on a bus, hurtling down Bondi Road, past the tattoo parlours and whole-foods stores, the charcoal chicken shops, and the beauticians advertising three Botox injections for $99.

Stan taps Carmel's arm and pegs two fingers over his nose.

Carmel nods. Extends her pinkie in the direction of the teenage boy with greasy hair and a t-shirt that says Dumb is Fun.

It's him. He's the one with the body odour.

Stan shakes his head. Inclines it towards the older guy in front. Faded flannel shirt and the bobbled nose of an experienced drinker. Carmel shrugs. Stan makes a wave motion with his hand, reminding her of their 1984 cruise around the Adriatic where an older American man, a history teacher, sat at their table every night and he had the most terrible . . . and the way he . . . and then he'd . . . oh, it was hilarious. Too hard to explain. You just had to be there.

Silently, Stan leans into her shoulder and Carmel covers her mouth to stifle a laugh.

At least they still have this. Their own private Auslan of nudges, nods and winks. Forty-six years of marriage not erased entirely. Not yet.

The bus stops outside a vegan pizzeria and Stan looks out the window. 'Where are we going again?'

'Sculptures. You remember?'

It's their yearly tradition, not that she writes it into her calendar. Just lets the seasons do their work. The soapy jasmine. The soft, purple rain from the jacaranda. Then, she knows. Time for their annual pilgrimage to the eastern beaches.

'Oh, yes. Sculptures.' Stan nods. 'I remember now.' Brow furrowed, fingers in a fist on his knee, he stares out the window looking for clues.

More knee-high socks and SLR cameras hop on the bus and the driver waits for them to sit before careering out into the traffic again.

Stan looks around at Carmel. 'Where are we going today?' Like a child on a holiday. Are we there yet?

Carmel clears her throat, swallows the dismay. Takes his hand and squeezes.

'It's alright. We'll be there soon.'

It's 9:30am and Mark's Park is almost empty, save for the seagulls wheeling about the sky like spent sandwich wrappers.

But there are the sculptures, of course, so still and mighty against a backdrop of restless ocean. Even under overcast skies, the effect of the momentous gathering—this corroboree of art—is dazzling, and breath stalls in Carmel's throat for the beauty of it all. Where to look first? At that neon-green shoot, fibre-glass perhaps, stretching high above the ground like Jack's beanstalk? Or that monolithic lump of sandstone, like the entrance to a cave leading to nothing but sea and sky?

Stan walks towards the stone monolith and reads the little square sign on the grass. 'Woman Walking. Number 22.'

Carmel follows beside him, runs her hand over the base. 'Looks like sandstone but it doesn't feel like it.'

Stan looks up between the great cleave in the rock. 'I think it's a vulva.'

Vulva? Carmel pretends she hasn't heard, checks to see no one else has. The crowd is already starting to build.

'I'll go and get a programme. You stay here.' She leaves Stan to contemplate the sandstone gash and heads to the merchandise tent where a small queue has formed.

Carmel has her ten dollars ready to go and cannot help but sigh as person after person shuffles about in their wallet, seemingly surprised that payment is expected even though the signage states it quite clearly: Programmes $10.

The woman in front of her, a mother, pushes her pram to the front of the queue.

'Ten dollars thanks,' says the young woman selling the booklets.

The mother pats her pockets. Rifles in her handbag. Her child is glued to a tiny screen making jarring noises that Carmel recognises as Dora the Explorer.

Thank God her grandchildren are past that stage.

'Sorry, the credit card was in my pocket.' The mother pats again, to be sure. 'Must be in my phone case.' She leans down to the child. 'Now, Rennie, sweetie, Mummy just needs to borrow her phone for a moment.'

The woman's voice is sugar-syrup and Carmel shifts weight. She cannot leave Stan for long, not with those steep slopes, just beyond the sculptures, that fall away to nothing but rocks and hungry seas.

Carmel inches forward and clears her throat as the mother fusses. 'Excuse me, but my husband is waiting and he's not well so would you mind if I just—'

The mother unfurls to full height. Lioness mode. Or is it cobra?

Something animal.

'Well, I have a child,' she snaps. 'And I don't appreciate your passive-aggressive tone.' The child starts to wail. 'Now look what you've done.' She douses him in kisses. 'Shush, Rennie-sweetie. Nearly there, darling.'

She hands over the credit card, gives the phone back to the child and wheels away without looking back.

'Sorry for the wait,' says the young woman in the booth.

'Not your fault,' says Carmel, clutching tightly to her ten dollars to calm the angry tremble in her fingers. What has so enraged her? It's just a silly young mother, after all. A mother who named her child after a heartburn treatment!

She breathes and hurries back to the rock sculpture.

There is no Stan and the park is busy now. So many cameras and phones that Carmel can almost feel the buzz of images making their way into the iCloud.

At last she finds him at the edge of the path, gazing down the coastline at the cataract-riven milkiness of the ocean and the cemetery two headlands away dotted with crosses. Last year, they saw a whale here. Hopefully that is what Stan is remembering.

'I thought I'd lost you.' She touches his arm gently so as not to frighten him out of his reverie.

He regards her and unfamiliarity fleets over his face before it is replaced with a smile. Frail synapses connecting. 'Thought I'd done a runner, eh?' He tucks her hand under his elbow. 'You can't get rid of me that easily.' He points down onto the beach below. 'I just saw a fox down there, you know.'

'What? Down on the sand?'

He nods and she squints in the direction of this finger. A fox in this place? This coastal suburbia where rows of window-eyed concrete mansions sit in dress circle formation like an unblinking audience for the ocean.

'I don't think so, Stan. Probably just a dog.'

'It was a fox.' He drops her hand. 'Don't you believe me?'

A delusion? Hallucination? Just go along with what he says, the doctor advised her. You'll only upset him.

'Come over to this one,' she says lightly. 'It's the Charge of the Light Horse at Beersheeba' She forces a smile through the quiver in her cheeks. 'Isn't it amazing?'

He stands before the stampeding herd, freeze-framed in steel. How has the artist done that? Captured the chaos and trauma of war with nothing but poles and sheets of rusty metal.

'It's incredible,' says Stan.

'I don't know how they do it,' says Carmel.

Stan steps in closer. 'You know, at the end of the war, a lot of the soldiers shot their own horses.'

She turns to him. 'Really? How awful.' 'Better than letting them rot away in Egypt.'

'But the Egyptians might have used them. Cared for them.'

Stan gently shakes his head. He thinks her naïve, she can tell. 'The soldiers felt it was merciful.'

She looks him in the eye. 'I think it cruel.'

They leave the horses and meander slowly down the cliff-top walk. Past the joggers and the surfers, the tourists and the school kids holding mobile phones to their noses like a third eye.

Stan and Carmel stop in front of a shiny, mirror-like sculpture, labelled Narcissus, and Carmel attempts an arty, ironic photo of them looking at their reflections.

She'll print it later and paste it to the visual calendar on the fridge where she keeps a record of everything they've done for the month, as a way of helping Stan remember. Sometimes, when he goes for the milk, Carmel catches him looking at it in wonder.

Was that really me in the Blue Mountains last week? Since when did I enjoy picnics in the Botanic Gardens? In and out, he peers, like a child discovering its hand.

Carmel offers to take a photo for some Japanese tourists standing before a model of three surfers that looks solid from front-on but nearly transparent from the side. They decline and produce a stick that extends from their phones like a robot arm.

'How ingenious,' says Stan, hands on hips.

'Yes, you never have to talk to anyone ever again.'

They walk slowly. Adjectives from fellow walkers float toward them on the breeze.

Shiny, isn't it . . . So beautiful . . . Deep, very deep.

Halfway down, there is a set of small, but highly detailed tribal figures. The program says they are made from sand and clay by artists of the South Pacific and the idea is to let the wind and spray take its toll.

Carmel points out where decay has set in, the frame of the figures poking through. Nothing but chicken wire.

They're nearly on the beach now and the sun is above them. Hot, especially for spring. It's been an age since Sydney's last decent rain. They retreat to the browned grass where there are yet more sculptures and a brand-new Hyundai, all shiny chrome and buffed- up wheels. A sales person with a ponytail and a corporate base-

ball-cap stands guard.

Stan points at the car. 'What's that sculpture called, then?' He smiles and pretends to look in his program.

They unwrap the sandwiches. Cheese and lettuce for her, chicken and avocado for him.

'You know, when I was a kid, I nearly died out there.' Stan munches slowly.

'You never told me that.' She looks at him, carefully. 'Got caught in a rip and it was like a freight train.' 'Who was with you?'

'Oh, Mum and Dad were somewhere. It was the fifties, you know. We didn't come here much.'

'How terrifying.' She finishes the sandwich and dusts the crumbs from her lap. 'I can't imagine.'

'It was the helplessness of it all. Completely at the mercy of the current.' He scrunches up the Glad Wrap. 'Awful.'

After lunch, Stan lies down. Hat propped over his face like a tent.

In minutes he is snoring.

Carmel takes up her book. Hours pass. The beach is in lull. 3pm, so, the school kids have gone and the tourists too. Carmel feels her eyes drooping. She lets the book fall closed. Closes her eyes briefly, then opens.

There, over there. A flash of something orange. Bushy tail. Elfin ears. Pinched nose.

It looks at her, twitching. Head at the angle of question.

Carmel sits up. She does not know what to do, who to tell, whether to wake Stan.

She touches him gently. 'Stan, wake up.' He is groggy, eye-rubbing. 'What is it?'

'I saw it. The fox. You were right, it's over there.'

She looks back to the bushes but the fox is gone. No orange tail. No darting eyes. Nothing.

'What are you talking about?' Stan is on his elbows. His eyes appraise her.

'That fox you saw from the cliff, it was real. It was there a second ago.' Carmel points to the bushes and Stan's gaze follows her finger.

'What fox?'

She clutches his elbow. 'You saw it, Stan. You did.'

His smile is thin. His eyes, pitying. Disappointed. A look she knows.

'I'm afraid you've lost me.' He lies down and closes his eyes, the setting sun throwing shadows, long and wide. 'You've completely lost me,' he murmurs.

Suffering is Universal

Jean Flynn

Third Prize

We're coming in with the shopping, me and the kids. I have Keely on my left hip and two bags in my right hand, knuckles clenched white. I tell Jett to wait on the porch, out of the drizzle, but he stays squatting by the front gate, poking at something in the weeds. There are eight bags all together: four trips from the car to the house, one week's worth of groceries. Keely starts whimpering as I shut the boot – her dummy's fallen into the gutter – and then I see Mariah's front door open, and out springs her red polka-dot umbrella. I walk up the path towards our house, wiping the dummy on my pants, jiggling Keely.

'Shh sh sh sh shhhh.'

Mariah raises the umbrella and there she is: porcelain skin and ash blond curls and lips like a ripe strawberry.

'Jett!' I shout.

Mariah looks over and smiles. Her dark green fingernails match her tights.

'Morning,' I say, hoiking Keely further up my side. I get a whiff of shit.

Mariah waves, bends into the rain and heads out of her gate and up the footpath. I wonder how long it takes to get her hair like that.

Jett runs to the porch and falls against the groceries. Oranges tumble down the steps and settle in the wet grass.

I look at my face in the mirror. It's the bags that I hate the most. The crow's feet are okay, not too bad yet, but the bags. I touch the puffy grey skin. Keely cries out and Jett runs into the bathroom.

'I didn't mean to do it!' he says, eyes wide.

We go into the lounge room, where Keely is lying on the floor, limbs thrashing like an upside-down beetle. I pick her up and kiss her salty face.

'What happened?' I say to Jett.

He clamps his teeth together and makes a quiet grunting sound. 'Come on, use your words.'

'She falled off the couch,' he says slowly, pressing his body against my legs. 'What a silly duffer.'

I watch Mariah arrive home. From where I'm sitting I can see right across our front yard and into hers. She walks with purpose, shoul- ders back. Jett is half a metre from the TV, legs crossed, mouth open. Keely is asleep on my chest, and if I move she'll wake up. I stroke her forehead and hum something my own mother used to hum to me.

'I want beetroot sandwiches for tea,' Jett announces.

I go to open the can but the ring pull isn't there. I flip the can over.

No ring pull.

'What's wrong, Mum?' he asks, one finger up his nose. 'We just have to go next door.'

Mariah is wearing a tie-dyed maxi dress. Her movement is gentle, like a dance. I ruin the choreography with a lurch forward, a thrust of beetroot can.

'D'you have a can opener?' I say.

'Mum can't find the pull ring,' says Jett, hands behind his back like a sergeant major.

Mariah smiles, first at Jett, and then at Keely. 'Of course I do,' she says. 'Come in.'

The house smells like an Indian restaurant. Jett charges up the hallway, arms out so that his fingertips brush against the floral wallpa- per. The kitchen is bright and cool.

'Is that dog food?' Jett asks, pointing to the bowl near the back door.

'It's for my cat, Charm,' Mariah says, opening a drawer.

There are pot plants on the microwave, the windowsill, the shelf above the sink. Stuck to one wall is a large print of the cross-legged Buddha, with 'KARMA' written underneath.

'My mum has a baby in her tummy,' says Jett, taking off one of his gumboots and tipping some tan bark onto the lino.

'Does she?' says Mariah, handing me the can opener.

I put chopped banana on the highchair tray and Keely says, 'Ba ba ba ba ba.'

'I want angles,' Jett says, pointing at his beetroot sandwich. 'Triangles.'

'Try angles.'

I cut the sandwich diagonally across, slice the crusts off and eat them.

'Where's Mariah's dad?' says Jett. 'You mean her husband?'

He chews with his mouth open and tips his head to one side. 'I guess she doesn't have one.'

We look at Keely, stuffing banana into her mouth and kicking her legs.

'Big guts!' Jett says.

The next morning I put on The Wiggles and google Buddhism.

I find out that:

- suffering is universal
- the cause of suffering is desire
- reincarnation is about energy transference but not souls
- all actions have consequences.

Jett stands up to sing Hot Potato. The yellow Wiggle is the only woman. I wonder if she is suffering. I wonder if she will become a yellow Labrador after she dies, or a canary.

I see Mariah arrive home. Sometimes she only works half days. She's wearing a long pink skirt, mauve singlet and a floppy straw hat. I am folding the washing while Keely is asleep. Jett is rolling marbles down toilet roll tubes.

'Pee-ooh!' he exclaims, as they come out the end and bounce onto the couch. 'Pee-ooh! Pee-ooh!'

Sometimes Mariah works from home. I see clients arrive – mostly middle-aged women – and leave an hour later. Can they hear our chaos, I wonder, while they're getting the knots in their shoulders pressed flat? Does Mariah play whale sounds and Enya to drown out the stamping and screaming and constant call of 'Mu-um!'?

'Why you doing that?' Jett asks, as I apply orange lacquer to my fingernails.

'Don't you like it?' I say.

'It's stinky!' He puts his face right next to my hands and scrunch- es up his nose.

Keely's in the high chair gobbling mandarin segments. When all ten fingers are done I blow on them.

'Are you cooling them off?' Jett asks.

I ruin the first two fingernails an hour later doing the dishes. Another chips when I drag a load of washing out of the machine. At dinnertime I look at the carrots in the fridge then decide to defrost some old bolognaise instead.

My lower back is sore. I don't know if it's the baby or carrying Keely or something else. I wish I had an hour free to lie on Mariah's massage table and close my eyes and have my flesh pummelled.

'When are we taking back the open canner?' says Jett, driving his Matchbox car along my arm.

'Let's go now,' I say, scooping Keely up onto my hip.

Mariah answers the door in a satin dressing gown. Her hair is wet. 'I'm sorry,' I say. 'To interrupt.'

'Is your cat here?' asks Jett.

Mariah holds her dressing gown closed and bends over. 'Yes,' she says. 'Would you like to see her?'

We go through to the kitchen, me still clasping the can opener. 'Charm,' sings Mariah. 'Here puss.'

The grey cat winds itself around her bare legs and Jett laughs. Keely wriggles to get down.

The kitchen is smaller than ours but lighter. Outside, in the backyard, the ground is covered with leaves the colour of sunset.

'Do you give Charm milk on a saucer?' says Jett, patting the tip of her tail.

'She just drinks water,' says Mariah, smiling.

'If I had a cat I would call him Mister Meow, but we can't have any pets 'cause Mum orready has enough people to look after.'

There is only one magnet on the fridge: Choose life, be vegan. 'Maybe when you're older, buddy,' I say. 'Come on.' Keely squeals

and kicks as I lift her up off the floor. 'Say goodbye.'

When I'm tucking Jett in that evening he says, 'Mum, where's Mariah's baby?'

'She hasn't got one,' I say, wiping his fringe to one side. 'Yes she has. In the photo.'

'What photo?' 'On the table.' 'In the kitchen?'

'No, where you go in.' 'Near the front door?'

'Yes. Where's that baby? Is it in bed?' 'I don't know. Maybe.'

When everyone is asleep I google veganism.

I find out that:

- tempeh is a good meat alternative
- tofu can be used to make dip
- even honey is off-limits.

I wonder if Aldi sells tempeh.

I go next door to see if Mariah has any soy sauce. The recipe wants me to marinate the tofu, and I only have oyster sauce, which is defi- nitely made of oysters and would therefore defeat the purpose.

There's hardly any left in the bottle, but Mariah insists that I take it.

'Really, it's fine,' she says, holding it out.

I glance in at the hall table and see the photo that Jett must have

been talking about. The picture is of Mariah holding a baby. They have the same rosebud lips, the same dimpled cheeks. The baby would be about six months, maybe a bit older. Mariah's looking at the camera, but the baby is looking at her.

'I'm marinating tofu,' I say.

'Toe foo is yucky,' Jett declares, pushing a piece off his fork.

'Keely likes it,' I say, scraping his leftover cubes onto the high- chair tray.

'Keely likes everything. Even cat food.'

There's rain coming—the sky is dark and the air feels damp—and spiders begin taking refuge inside the house. I take the Mortein out of the high cupboard.

'There's one!' says Jett, pointing at the wall above the front door. 'Stand back,' I tell him. 'And keep Keely out of the way.'

I point the can at the small huntsman and spray. The poison smells like mixed lollies and nail polish remover. I open the front door as the spider drops, paralysed, to the floor.

'Mum!' says Jett. 'Look!'

There are two black spiders on the porch ceiling. 'Stay there,' I say.

I step out, one hand stiff around the Mortein. Keely squeals and tries to crawl towards me. 'Have you got her?' I say.

'Do it, Mum,' Jett says, arms around his sister's tummy.

I take aim just as Mariah comes out of her front door. The spray cloud is immense and I am lost in the fog for a moment. As the spiders lose their grip and fold up into balls I see Mariah look over then look away. She doesn't smile, or wave. Her face looks slightly pinched.

'Pee-ooh, pee-ooh!' says Jett, a satisfied grin on his little face. 'Killed! Killed!'

When I shove the Mortein back in the cupboard I notice that only my pinky fingernail is still unblemished and think, well, all actions have consequences.

The following week I have to take Keely for her 12-month check-up. She strains backwards as I try to do up her seatbelt.

The maternal health nurse is pleased.

'This baby is thriving,' she says, looking at the scales.

'What does thriving mean?' asks Jett, stacking coloured wooden blocks into a tower.

'Fat,' I say.

'Mum-um-um,' says Keely, reaching for me. 'Because of all that toe foo,' says Jett.

'Yes. Our very own little Buddha.'

Red Belly

Jane O'Sullivan

Highly Commended

Jem lived in the caravan and the red belly black snake lived under- neath it. They understood each other well enough. Most of the time it stayed out of sight and, in return, he pushed bits of sausage out the tiny window above the kitchenette. Not too many though, the world didn't need fat snakes.

Still, he took care. He hit the lino hard of a morning, swinging himself down from his narrow bunk. Then he'd creak open the door and stand with his black and two sugars, looking out at the world and giving it time. Only then would he lower himself onto the wooden steps. They were prefab pine ones that he'd got from Bunnings several months after a storm had blown the old plastic stepstool away. They made a dark portal to the underneath. He trusted his snake but he never went down those stairs quickly.

Sometimes, when he was standing with his feet in the sand and his line in the ocean, he'd think about googling it. Snake poison red belly how long? The road was pretty good now. They'd paved in nearly all of it. But it was still a fair forty minute drive to town. It could get messy. But he never got around to finding out for sure. Somehow, by the time he'd got his rod and bucket back on his four wheel drive, the thought had always slipped from him like a fish.

Besides, there was enough to do already. He'd had to sort that step, hadn't he? And now there was the rust. The caravan had only meant to do for a couple of months. 'Sure. This one,' he'd told the caretaker on his quaddie, letting his rough, quick-beat anxiety march him through the decision. That was four years ago now. He'd bought a tarp a while back, and a rope to tie it down, just to tide him over. It fluttered and slapped in the wind. (And there was always wind here, by the sea.)

And then there was his mother. She'd learned to text, because he never answered when she called. Sometimes, when he could manage it, he'd ring her back. 'What's news?' she'd ask. 'Nothing,' he'd say. 'You?'

She didn't really understand his reticence—she liked talking— but she knew how to move through it now. She no longer left gaps. And Jem liked her reports. They were circuitous and straight to the point and all the things he could not be because he never went anywhere.

Then he ruined it. He'd driven home with three silver-scaled trophies strung to his roo bar, a victory worth celebrating. He'd seen her message and he'd pressed the little green phone icon underneath it. But instead of telling her about the fish, he told her about the snake. 'I have a snake,' he said. 'Under the caravan.' Before he could even

be startled by what he'd done, her squeal had leaped the gulf from Sydney to Bobbin Heads, from his phone to his ear, and had shook the thin skin drum with a mother's grip. He yelped. 'Jesus, mum.'

She stopped herself and breathed. 'Well, get rid of it, you dolt.

You're not bloody Tarzan.'

'Did Tarzan like snakes?' he said. 'I never read that book.'

'No one's read that book,' she spat. 'No one likes snakes. No one sane, anyway.'

'I didn't say I did,' he said, feeling the agitation kick in like a double shot of coffee. Could the snake feel the vibrations of his voice through the caravan floor? Did it know what that meant? His mum sighed, low and heavy, like a diesel engine changing gears. 'Do you want me to call someone?' she asked. 'Tell me what kind of snake and I'll call someone.'

'No,' he said, fighting the pull. 'I'll deal with it. It's not a problem.' But the snake had heard.

The next day (because, of course, he could do nothing that after- noon after talking to his mum), he slowly shuffled around his caravan as his tea got cold and the dawn seeped in through the blinds. It was only after he told himself there was no point missing the fish, that he could deal with it later, that he was able to unlatch the door. The caravan groaned as he stepped out. He was across the brick pavers and nearly at the car when he saw it. The snake was right there, curled on the inside of the front passenger side tyre. The high lift meant he could see it clearly. There was no reason for it to be there, though. There were no sunbeams for it there. Nor was there any cover. Besides, if it wanted to hide it would still be under the caravan where it was low and dank and dark and the birds couldn't see it.

The kookas were game around here. Big, too.

He felt anger first. Did it want to get itself killed? Then resentment. How was he meant to get out now? Was he meant to not go fishing? Jem walked slowly around the four wheel drive. He pulled at the driver's side door. He squatted and peered under. No movement. So he took a giant step and hauled himself into the cab.

It still smelt like Lou a little bit, his old boxer. Could the snake smell that, he wondered, with its tongue? But then, his car smelt like lots of things, fish mostly, and had done for some time. The snake had already had plenty of time to learn that. He rocked the key in the barrel, a gentle, practiced sequence of wrist movements, and the old beast ticked over. The engine rumbled. He sat there, his hand still resting on the key, feeling the shake through his feet and his arse and all the way up to his outstretched arm. Lou had been a good dog.

He knew it was a cliché. Everyone thinks their dog is a good dog. But Jem knew the truth: some dogs are not good dogs. Some dogs are dickheads. And if you luck out, you still have to keep it unless you happen to be just as much of a dickhead as your dog. Life was tricky that way.

He'd managed to do things for Lou all the time. He hadn't even minded. Not the vet. Not the tablets. Not even picking up her poo and feeling her body warmth travelling through the thin plastic and into his hand. It had been easier doing things for her than for himself.

He left the door open and let the car burble as the sun crept into the day. He imagined the engine rumbles travelling into the sandy earth and back up into that little red belly. Move on, move on. This monster truck is coming to life.

Then he saw Mug looking out his slot window, a thin strip of rolling eyes and pissed off lip. Mug did not like being awake before nine. Jem rested his foot on the steel sidestep and stretched himself back onto the dirt. He squatted again. He felt the trace of an ant clambering across his foot at its crazy firesale pace. He looked. The snake's head still rested on the coil of its own body. Its eye seemed to look straight at him. 'Go on, get out of here,' he said, waving his hand uselessly in front of him.

Mug was out now, standing on his front step in a pair of bright hibiscus boardies. His white chest hair curled over a torso that had once been keg shaped but was now up to barrel.

'Car trouble?' he called out. Jem shook his head and pointed under the carriage. 'Bloody snake's called shotgun on me.' He said it with what he hoped was just the right amount of surprise. Mug looked disappointed but he padded across the scrappy grass to look. 'Yep,' he said. 'Looks like a red belly.'

Jem pretended to consider this, then agreed. 'I thought it'd move if it felt the car start up.'

'Doesn't look like it,' he said. 'I'll get the shovel.'

Jem lifted off his heels but stopped before he took a step. He looked at Mug across the bonnet. Then he saw Mug's hips swivel and his barrel chest start to follow. He felt the tide start to take him. 'Can you even do that?' he started.

'What, with a shovel? Yeah,' said Mug. 'Slow, though. Gotta creep up on them slow.'

'No, I mean . . . ,' stuttered Jem. 'Killing it. I don't know. Isn't it endangered? Aren't there rules?'

Mug raised his arms and swung them around in a questioning arc. Jem followed it. The caravan park was quiet except for the rumble of the four wheel drive and usual chatter of the birds. All the serious fish- ermen had left an hour ago. It was just them.

Jem felt everything fall in, as though a king tide had swallowed him. It wouldn't let him find the words.

Mug took his silence and gathered it up and went to get his shovel. Jem heard him scuff back onto his lot. He heard the creak of his old tradie tool chest. Metal banged on metal. A green bird shot overhead, calling out like a dying cat.

He walked in a wide circle around the car. He came in quietly, crouching down a metre or two from the snake. 'You gotta move,' he told it. He stood, and he stamped his foot, then again and again. Dust rose up. The snake stayed still. Its nictating membrane dropped and lifted in a tiny, transparent blink. Was it even able to get moving? Was it warm enough? When it came down to it, he knew bugger all about snakes.

He heard Mug's footsteps behind him, and then the blade of the shovel thunk into the ground, then the sound of Mug sucking in another breath. Jem turned to face him. The sun made his chest hair glow like silver armour. 'Alright, Jemmy, let's be done with it.'

Jem felt the weight of the water. He kicked. 'Maybe I could borrow your shovel?'

Mug's eyebrows shot up. Jem reached out his arm, palm up. A universal symbol. Mug, in return, offered his own. He stepped back- wards, giving him space, and rested his hands on hips. But Jem didn't feel like performing. He curled his fingers around the handle, worn smooth but riven with cracks, and waited. Mug raised his palms in mock concession and swung his great white shark of a body back towards his lot. 'Drop it back when you're done,' he threw over his shoulder. The sound wobbled in the air, but before the words could hit Jem the black cockatoos cawed through them and broke them to pieces.

Jem looked back at the snake, and sat down.

Excess Baggage

Tanya Vavilova

Highly Commended

The teenage girl and her grandma sit at the kitchen table eating kasha and drinking Nescafé. Julie thinks Olga looks like a butter- nut pumpkin, squat and sturdy, her hair a light orange, long faded. She blends into the décor, like the wallpaper or stove, a permanent fixture in this Moscow apartment for almost forty years.

Olga has been watching the news, all day, every day, following the situation in Ukraine. She's upset by what she sees and is thankful her government is doing everything it can to help. The Russian convoy has been trying to deliver supplies for days.

Julie doesn't need to watch the news, she's sure her grandma's got it wrong. The same events are reported differently back home. She grew up with James Bond and cartoons whose villains were always called Igor.

Olga gently opens the window letting the chilly air ruffle the curtains. The thermostat is set for the entire apartment block at the beginning of winter and once the weather warms up the tenants crack open their windows. It's just the way things are.

Resting her elbows on the tablecloth, Julie stares out at the milky sky. She listens to her grandma chew and the classical music playing on the radio. She thinks it's Stravinsky but is too shy to ask.

After she scoops up the last apricot in her kasha, she collects the cups and plates and squeezes out the lurid green liquid for the washing up. Funny, they use the Fairy brand here too.

Olga lives at the second last stop of the Sokol'nicheskaya line. The flat is on the ninth floor of a concrete tower, in a row of identical blocks, grey and mint green. Olga feels like a beetle in a matchbox. People should not live like this—all bunched up, anonymous. She still keeps the old papers for her family's home. They haven't meant anything for a long time.

Every time Julie swings open the heavy entrance door the smell of socks and old books surprises her. She holds her breath. The hall is musty, the windows never opened. On the left, a row of neat grey letterboxes gives her the stink-eye. How long since the peach-colour- ed garbage chutes were used? She knows not to comment; knows that people are lucky to live here.

Julie, her grandma calls from her room, come here. Ok, babushka.

It's Ukraine. Julie sighs.

She reluctantly leaves the warmth of the kitchen to sit on the edge of her grandma's bed.

Olga sits with her hands clasped, her eyes big and sad. The politi- cian in the red blazer is talking about the atrocities, pointing the finger at the international community.

The volume's too high for Julie. She can't make out the words.

When the sun is low on the horizon, they usually read, each in their own room, their doors flung open. Halfway through a chapter, Julie hears the shuffle of her grandma's slippers. Again they will attempt conversation.

Can I come in? her grandma asks. Of course.

Olga sinks into the stripy brown sofa. What are you reading? A book by Tim Winton.

Who is Tim Winton?

Julie's Russian is scratchy, hard for Olga to understand. Why didn't they teach the girls to speak Russian? She'd bought both Julie and her sister Russian alphabet books when they were small.

He's a famous Australian writer, Julie says. It's about two families, the Pickles—Ogurets—and the Lambs. What's the word? She bleats.

Yagnyat? Da, da.

Such funny names! Olga laughs.

And they live in a house in Perth split down the middle like a watermelon.

Perth?

Julie traces the map of Australia in the air. Our famous poet is Pushkin, Olga says.

Julie listens politely as her grandma recites The Water Nymph. After a while, Olga gets up. Do you want tea?

Olga pads to the kitchen and looks out at the silvery sky while the kettle boils. A raven flits from branch to branch. She pours the hot water over her day-old bitter brew. Old habits of conservation. Adds a slice of lemon and a little sugar.

She puts the tea tray down and stretches out on her single bed. Suddenly, she's very tired. The proud birch and maple trees peer in through the window. Thick foliage of a verdant green. Quiet relief.

Having offered to cook lunch for her grandma, Julie walks to the grocer on the corner. A drift of smiling pigs adorns the entrance. Like Margaret Atwood's spliced pigoons.

She pushes open the heavy glass door, holding it open for a teenage boy with a walking stick.

It's warm inside, no air-con.

Walking past the bruised fruit in the crates, Julie stops to gawk at the bright packages and tins. A whole row of bottled orgurets!

What's the conversion rate? Forty-five roubles to the dollar. She counts out the correct change, smiles at the cashier.

When she reaches the ninth floor, her grandma is ready, holding open the door.

Bozhe moy, bozhe moy! They're very heavy. Give them to me. Australian kids are very strong.

You found the Danish butter? Olga asks. She'd worried it had disappeared with the sanctions.

I got three packs. Too many.

While the television murmurs in Olga's room, Julie arranges the ingredients on the bench top. Tomatoes. Onions. Beef mince. Spag Bol is one meal she knows how to cook.

She loves the smell of frying onions, the way they turn pearly.

The mince sizzling and spitting. She opens the window a sliver.

After a while, her grandma shuffles into the kitchen. Is it ready? Soon, Julie says. I'll call you.

Her grandma is used to living on her own, eating whenever she likes.

After a few mishaps—she slices her thumb, drops the hunk of cheese on the floor—Julie serves up the Spag in white and blue Gzhel bowls and sets them on the table.

Olga sits in her usual spot by the window. Do you like it? Julie asks hopefully.

Not for me. Too spicy.

Julie wonders what flavours her grandma is referring to. There's no chilli in the sauce.

Days and days before her granddaughter arrived, Olga made up the room with matching sea-blue sheets and blankets and stocked the fridge with delicacies—imported cheese, a red and gold tin of caviar.

On the first night, she'd asked Julie if she still liked sugar-coated cranberries

What? Julie had asked.

I bought a box of sugar-coated cranberries. You used to love them. When?

When you lived here with your parents and sister. I was four, babushka. How could I remember?

Olga carried the box into her bedroom and, while Julie slept off the jetlag, she ate the cranberries in front of the flickering TV.

Too fast, babushka, Julie says. You speak too quickly for me.

. . . the celebrations in the Red Square for Victory Day. My knees are bad, otherwise I'd go.

You can watch it on the television.

Putin, of course, will give a speech about Russia, her military capa- bilities, her hardy people . . . He's a very clever man.

The way her grandma says this confuses Julie. He understands the people.

Why are you talking like that? Julie demands. Like someone is listening through the wall?

Olga is silent.

No one is eavesdropping, babushka.

When they go sightseeing together, Olga takes extra care of her appear- ance. She conceals the scalloped scars on her neck with powder and picks out nice shoes. Her granddaughter has that careless beauty of the young and Olga knows she'd had it too. When she shows Julie photos of youth camps and field trips, her wedding day, Julie tells her she was stunning. They look alike and this makes Olga very, very happy.

A new department store has opened up near the station. Olga, with bad knees and high hopes, drags Julie there on a drizzly Tuesday. Julie knows she won't buy anything; she's brand conscious and choosy. Looking sideways at the puffy jackets and vests she can't bring herself to try anything on.

What about this? Her grandma points to a navy jacket with a fur trim.

Too warm for Sydney. A hat?

Not for me.

Don't you like anything here? her grandma asks.

They're beautiful but not for me. Let's go?

Olga tries to hide her disappointment.

One evening, Julie hears her grandma rummaging in her wardrobe; a wall-length structure, dark wood, cavernous. Things vanish inside: clothes, photo albums, letters, figurines. She knows her grandma has a collection of expensive porcelain dolls behind the glass, compensa- tion for a childhood marred by war.

Here, have this, Olga says, pushing a handbag into Julie's hands. It's brown Italian leather, expensive-looking.

My cousin gave it to me. I won't use it. Do you want it? Thank you, Julie says. She knows to refuse would be rude. Finally, her granddaughter likes something!

Wait, I have one more thing, she says. Julie holds her breath.

Her grandma pulls out a bronze statue of Pushkin. Our national poet, she announces.

It's the sheen and size of a small saucepan.

Julie looks at the bust. What is she going to do with him? Take it.

She is surprised by its weight and almost drops the father of literature.

To go with your Winton, Olga says. She starts to put all the things back in the cupboard. She won't let Julie help; only she herself knows where everything goes. She has so little in the world.

Julie examines her tummy in the shower. Round like blini and potatoes. The top button of her jeans always undone. She misses her mum and her friends. Sleepovers and stakeouts. She loves her grandma but it's all jumbled up. Like a garage sale. Some feelings a bit rusty, misplaced.

They share a pot of tea in the kitchen, and turn the radio up. Olga gets a dusty photo album out. Look, she says, that's you and your sister.

Which is which?

You're the one with the dimples.

They're only two years apart.

More tea?

Julie pours steaming, brown liquid into both cups.

Who's that?

That is your uncle Boris. He was a priest too.

They look through the album, refilling th eir te acups, as th e su n dips below the horizon and the neighbours start coming home.

On the morning Julie is due to fly out, they walk to the corner of the block. Olga's knees are too weak to go further today. She looks at her granddaughter, pleased to see she has put some flesh on her boneJus.lie adjusts her backpack. Don't watch too much news, she says.

Terrible what's happening in Ukraine. Da, da.

Send me a message when you land. Okay, babushka.

Love you.

Julie looks at her shoes. I'll come back soon. Olga wants to believe her.

On her way to the station, Julie passes the red-bannered department store. A little girl and her mother exit with a slim plastic bag. The girl is singing a pop song. Shakira?

Why didn't she let her grandma buy her the fur coat? It would've been so easy. But she'd shaken her head, said no, and the two of them walked home in the drizzle.

The little girl shakes her hips and beams at Julie as they cross each other on the road.

At the airport check-in, Julie hoists her suitcase onto the conveyer built.

The woman with the painted eyebrows looks her over and says, two kilos over.

Julie goes through her suitcase. It's poor old Pushkin.

How much? she asks the attendant. Three thousand roubles.

Julie does a quick mental calculation. If you round up to fifty, one thousand roubles is $20 so three thousand roubles is $60.

She can't recite a single line of Pushkin's poetry. Pictures him in the airport trashcan, lying sideways, among bits of paper and plastic. Chewy stuck to his eye.

She hands over her bankcard. She will take him home.

The lady gives her a docket.

You can go through now, she says.

Postcard

Wayne Strudwick

Commended

It takes him three days to get to his father's funeral. There are delays and misconnections, a night spent in some airport lying twisted beneath blinking fluorescent, sleep deprived and tortured by noise, and then from Sydney he catches a Greyhound to Tamworth and transfers to a busted-up Denning, half-a-dozen on board, and rattles out to the western plains.

He looks out at the red soil country, at the flat paddocks of wheat stubble and myall trees, where bone-thin Herefords graze on the meager pickings. He still has the postcard he'd bought months ago in Switzerland, and he takes it out of his pocket and looks at the herd of Jerseys grazing in a meadow, thick grass to their flanks, snow-capped alps in the background. He turns the card over and reads his little quip about European cattle, about the privilege, the luxury. The card is stamped and addressed to his father. But he never sent it.

The grain silos of Cullabri appear in the distant shimmer. Just past the C20 sign he looks for the old rut road cutting through wire- grass south of the blacktop. The road leads to a set of double gates at the boundary fence and he can see that the gates have rusted and come off the hinges. He thinks about the chain and padlock latched between those gates when the bank foreclosed and took possession of the farm, and he remembers the men who came to move them off and lock the gates, those fat men in suits, obscene in those ridiculous suits with the heat and the dust all around, their faces red and dripping, swatting flies and cursing as they tried to loop the heavy chain through the wire mesh. It happened three years ago and the humiliation still gnaws into him. He slides the postcard back into his pocket.

The old bus hits the slats of the Warrener Creek Bridge and goes up over the levy and through the outskirts of Cullabri. Rusted bill- boards on the roadside. Population 3500. He looks at the wide empty streets and the gutted cars up the dirt laneways and he wonders where all the people are.

His sister is waiting at the post office, pacing the pavement. He takes his backpack from the overhead rack and gets off the bus.

'You realize the time?' she says. 'Not exactly in my control, Julie.'

They hesitate then hug briefly. She looks him up and down. 'Tell me you have a suit, Michael.'

'No I don't have a fucking suit.' 'Jeans and t-shirt, this is your plan?'

'I didn't plan to backpack in a suit, if that's what you mean.'

Her face is stamped with worry and malcontent. Was she 30 yet? She looked it. The last he knew she was tucked into a cozy suburban home with a husband, a kid and a kitchen under renovation.

'We'll go to Dad's and get you cleaned up at least,' she says, checking her watch. 'The funeral is in t-minus one hour.'

'T-minus? What, are we launching him into space?' 'How about some respect, Michael.'

He follows her to a yellow Barina with a baby-on-board sign stuck to the back window. He gets in and rolls down the window. The car smells of sour milk.

'How's your kid?' he says.

'My kid? My kid is fine. He's walking and talking.'

She'd named the kid Atticus. Atticus. Talk about loading it with expectation.

'Is that normal?' he says. 'I mean, like, how old is he?' 'Fourteen months.'

'So you still count in months?' She doesn't respond.

They arrive at the council flats on the western edge of town and he gets out and stands on the road. The hot wind gusts and a chip packet skids along the gutter.

'Where did it happen?' he says.

'Not far from where you're standing.'

He looks up and down the road. No cars, no people. He imagines his father lying on the road, marks of worry harrowed down his face, sun beating down on the black tar. Alone on the road.

'How does this happen?' he says, arms out, palms up. 'On this road? In this town?'

She shakes her head. She looks angry, and she turns away and walks toward the flats. Then she stops and faces him. 'Are you remotely upset that Dad passed away?' she says.

'Passed away?'

'Okay, that he died, that he was killed.'

'You'd prefer that I was crying? Is that what you want, Julie? You tell me what you want.'

'It's just some inconvenience for you, isn't it.'

He glares at her. 'Of course I'm upset,' he says.

She crosses the dead lawn and opens the door to their father's unit. He stays on the road and looks west and listens to the rising drone of a wheat lorry coming in from the scrub. He can't believe he was in Amsterdam just days ago, walking along the canal in strafing rain, news of his father seeping into him like something cold in his veins.

The unit is simple and neat. A table with placemats, a couch with cushions neatly stacked, a small kitchen with one bowl on the dish- rack. He visited once, not long after his father had moved in, when the bareness of the place, the feeling of loneliness, of desperation, drove him out. He only stayed two days.

'Have you tidied up?' he says. 'This is how I found it.'

There are pictures of Julie and the kid everywhere, on the fridge, on the table, on the mantelpiece, and there are pictures of his father with people he doesn't recognize, groups of people bunched together, grinning. Framed certificates hang on the wall, Bushfire Brigade, First Aid, Driving Instructor. His father had told him about the student drivers; they were girls mostly, girls he'd met while stacking shelves at Zumbo's FoodMart, and Michael remembers wanting to change the subject, wanting to get off the phone, because he didn't want to know about the teenage girls he was instructing or about the grocery shelves he was stacking.

On a small shelf by the lounge he spots a photo of himself from Cullabri High graduation. He's wearing a rented suit and a red bowtie and he looks awkward, looks like he wants to get away. At the edge of the frame is a hint of his mother's arm hooked through his own, her face cut from the scene.

He goes into the bedroom and slings off his backpack. There is a pile of books on the bedside table, Penguin Classics mostly and a Stephen King thriller, and it surprises him because he'd only known his father to read the Land newspaper; he had never seen him read a book. There is a diary in the pile and he takes it out and flicks through the pages. There is no commentary, no reflection, only work schedules, meetings and social engagements. Every day is filled with activity. Choir practice? He'd never heard his father sing.

He opens the wardrobe. The smell is familiar but the clothes are not. He holds this memory of his father as a farmer in filthy King Gees and Blunstones, as a man among machinery, crops and cattle. But in the wardrobe there are trousers and shirts neatly ironed, ties on a rack and shiny shoes in a line on the floor. He begins to wonder who his father had become. Who was this man with friends and hobbies, this town man with clean clothes and a tidy home? He stands before the clothes breathing in the smell of his father.

The feeling comes on quickly, catching him out, a strong downward tugging in his chest, his heart pounding, and it folds him over, drops him to the floor, and he curls up beneath the clothes and grabs his t-shirt and wrenches it up over his face.

Julie is standing in the doorway. 'What are you doing?' she says. 'Just give me a second will you.'

'Is there something wrong with you?'

He crawls out of the wardrobe, leans back against the bed and pulls the t-shirt away from his face. He bows his head, unable to look at her. 'It's just that he had this life, you know?' he says. 'This life that I

knew nothing about.'

'And whose fault is that, Michael?'

It takes everything in him not to scream at her. His breath comes shuddering out of him. 'I know it's my fault,' he says slowly, his teeth clenched.

She comes into the room, stands above him, an arm resting on her hip.

'I just didn't let him in,' he says. 'He embarrassed me.' 'Embarrassed?'

'Him losing the farm the way he did. Mum pissing off. All that. I

couldn't handle the shame of it.' He looks up at her. 'It's unforgiveable what I've done, Julie.'

'I'm not sure what you want me to say,' she says. 'Then just leave me alone.'

She sits on the end of the bed. 'Why do you always want to be left alone,' she says. 'Do you think it helps, being left alone?'

He pulls the shirt over his face. He can't stand looking at her. 'You just have to face up to it, Michael.'

'Face up to what?'

'I'll let you figure that out,' she says. 'I'll wait in the car.'

He opens the backpack and looks at the rolled up t-shirts and jeans, the wrinkled gortex, the beanie and gloves. The smell lifting off the clothes is sharp, a pungent stink of the unwashed traveler, and he pushes the backpack away and gets to his feet. He takes out a grey suit from the wardrobe and lays it on the bed. Then he selects a shirt and tie and a pair of black shoes. He undresses and shoves the old clothes into his backpack and then slips an arm into the cool linen of his father's crisp white shirt. He puts on the suit and laces the shoes. The clothes are too big for him, but he doesn't care. He finds a belt and hitches it round his waist and leaves the house.

It is a small graveside service. People come up and shake his hand; some hug him. He feels like a fraud, like he doesn't deserve their sorrow. He suffers through it. When it is over he notices two girls in Culla High uniforms talking softly at the back of the gath- ering. He walks up to them and introduces himself. One of the girls dabs her eye with a tissue.

'How did you know my father?' he says.

'He taught us to drive,' the girl with the tissue says. 'He was so nice to us. My Dad just swore at me and gave up. But your father was so patient, so kind. He was funny, too. He'd always make us laugh.'

'He was a really good teacher,' the other girl says. 'You were lucky to have a father like him.'

'Thankyou,' he says. 'Thankyou for telling me that.' He looks at these two young girls, no older than sixteen, both of them grieving for his father. 'I think you're the lucky ones,' he says.

He stands above the grave. He will place the postcard on the coffin as it is lowered into th e gr ound. He ha s pl anned th is fin al gesture since leaving Amsterdam, when he found the abandoned card in the bottom of his pack. His father would've liked what he'd written; it would've made him smile. He looks at the dates on the headstone, at the year 1999, and he thinks about these numbers rolling over to 2000 in just a few weeks. He knows he must change. The coffin begins its slow descent. He reaches into his pocket, but the postcard is not there. He has left it in the pocket of his jeans. He watches the coffin go down. He did not think it would go so deep.

Dachshunds on antidepressants

M.J. Reidy

Commended s

Your mother tells you that Gerry, her one year old dachshund, has been diagnosed with a mental illness. The behaviour therapist told her it was pretty serious.

'What sort of mental illness?' you ask.

'We're not sure yet. But there's definitely signs of anxiety.' She is silent for a while. You tell your mother that you read on Beyond Blue recently that one out of four Australians experience anxiety. Maybe it's the same with dogs. And the stats even higher for small dogs, like dachshunds, that wander through the world staring up at the sphinc- ters of Alsatians like the puckered mouths of old men.

'Perhaps it's normal, Mum. You think about it—Gerry is up against a world of much bigger, more aggressive dogs.'

'Mmm.' She sounds flat, a little depressed. 'Well, it's not your fault.'

'Oh, I know that,' she says quickly. 'They're going to put him on an antidepressant.' You roll your eyes so far back in your head that it hurts.

You indulge her for a while. 'So, what was Gerry's childhood like?'

'Well, this is the thing. We paid a lot of money for him and he was from a show breeder. I mean he won awards for the best show dog in Dubbo.' Your mother scoffs as if dogs of better breeding are impervious to mental illness; to anxiety.

You tell her that it was perhaps the pressure, the high expec- tations to perform. You imagine dog shows are equivalent to those creepy beauty pageants for six year olds in the U.S. It mustn't be easy for a dachshund to cope with that.

'Yes, perhaps,' she says and in the long silence that follows you can hear her brain ticking over, trying to psychoanalyse the whole thing.

'Maybe he was bullied by his brothers and sisters in the litter?' 'Mmm, yes. That's a very good point.'

'Or maybe,' you say, trying to keep your voice steady, 'maybe his mother was so wrapped up with her own life, with her own problems that she neglected him. Maybe he's never gotten over that.'

There is a long pause down the phone line.

'I think there's something in that,' she says. 'I'm going to send an email to the breeder, so I can get a sense of his family dynamics.'

For a joke you once nominated your mother and Archie—the other dachshund—for Dr Harry's show on TV. Dr Harry would meet with pet-owners, people desperate to cure their wayward whippets, cocka- toos that muttered cunt-cunt-cunt at the dinner table, cats that pissed on the couch.

Archie the dachshund was sick too for a while. Like Gerry. Neurotic. Anxious. Howling when a storm came and pacing up and down like a junkie looking for a hit. But then Gerry came along and she seemed to forget all about it.

Your mother tells you that every afternoon for the last seven days she has sat with Gerry out the front of Coles.

'Desensitisation, the dog behaviourist calls it. I have him on his lead and he gets liver treats for being good.'

'Right,' you say. 'Exposure therapy.'

'Ah, yes. Just like how they treat PTSD and trauma?' You know this because you were diagnosed with it years ago.

'Yes, exactly. I am gradually introducing him to people so that he doesn't bark or snap.' You think of Gerry and his biting and barking and wonder if it is a normal reaction to the world; to the tens of thou- sands of assholes that fill it up.

'Maybe there's nothing wrong with him, Mum. Maybe he's intu- itive. Clever. Maybe he's got a finely tuned nose that can pick up the scent of psychopaths and sociopaths?'

'Oh please,' she scoffs. 'He's a dog.' 'Mmm,' you say.

'I could write a book about this,' she says, trying to impress you because you are a writer.

'About what exactly?'

'Well, when I sit outside Coles with Gerry every afternoon lots of people come up to me. They say how beautiful Gerry is, comment on his beautiful coat. Complete strangers just sit down next to me and talk. Really open up. I feel a lot like Forrest Gump.'

'Well dog's are a good conversation starter. It breaks the ice.'

'Yes,' she says. 'It's rather lovely. It's nice just being out and amongst people again.'

'That's nice,' you add. Since your stepfather's back surgery and your mother's hip operation she seems a little lost and lonely—trips to Coles are as far as she can get.

You put on your best twangy American accent, determined to cheer her up. 'L-ife is l-ike a box of chocolates. Or a dachshund on ant-iii-depress-ants.'

She laughs, then stops. 'Actually, he's been very good,' she says, 'since he's been on those antidepressants.'

You ask her what she means by 'good.'

'Well he sleeps a lot. And he's stopped picking on Archie. And he actually seems to listen and obey me now.' You wonder if by obeying she means so comatosed he falls asleep in his food bowl or keels over like one of those fainting goats, mid-way through a game of ball.

'Well that's something, isn't it?' you say and hang up.

You wonder if your mother's rigorous discipline of Gerry is some sort of compensation for her lack of control over her own life, her ailing health.

You think about this a lot.

She used to swim two kilometres a day and play the banjo and the ukulele but now, at 68, there are signs of illness. Rheumatoid arthritis. Peripheral neuropathy. A sudden dropped foot, which means she can only walk with a crutch. Gnarled fingers that will not cooperate and allow her to clasp her own bra.

Your mother is tired. She has had enough. Sometimes she looks at your stepfather and you wonder if she wants a refund, some sort of exchange. She didn't sign up for this. Chronic pain. Medical appoint- ments that fill up their week. Their life was once filled with BBQs and cruises and that ubiquitous Asian noodle salad. It's been 40 years since your stepfather returned from Vietnam but he is continuing to fight a war. PTSD. Depression. Anxiety. That one sneaky wine that leads to a whole bottle. Back surgery, four knee replacements, a double heart bypass at aged 47.

And every time your mother or stepfather get another health scare, your mother drags Gerry out to the back reserve, yanking the leash tight. You can see the scene in your head: the bum bag of liver treats hanging like a colostomy bag at her waist, your mother taking ten paces back. *Sit Gerry. Stay*. Wait. One hand held out in front of her like a stop sign.

You can see Gerry blinking, tilting his head. Trying to under- stand why he has to sit so still. But you're pretty sure that stop sign is not meant for him at all – it's your mother's way of saying: *Make this ageing and illness stop! Sit, stay, heel, like an obedient dog at my feet.*

15 years ago.

After two years backpacking around the world you returned home to live with your mother and her new husband.

You sit at the dinner table as your mother waxes lyrical about the joys of Dyson vacuum cleaners and Egyptian cotton and what Kieran Perkins is going to do in his retirement.

'Perhaps he'll do sports psychology? Or become a coach?' You shrug. You really don't give a fuck.

After you finish dinner you watch your stepfather sit cross-legged on the floor cleaning the dachshund's teeth with chicken liver tooth- paste, staring at the dog's bared gums.

In order to cope—to not end up in hospital again with depres- sion—you pretend that you are a French au pair, named Jacquelyn, who has flown halfway around the world and somehow landed in this house with these strange people and their dogs.

During the week you work as a waitress in an Italian restaurant, serving people their half-strength soy lattes and almond friands. At the end of every shift you scull a triple-shot cappuccino, thinking of how exhausting all those repressed middle class people seem. Then you return home and do it all again—listening to conversations about Shane Warne and Ita Buttrose and how the Liberal party will pull the economy out of its slump. You sit there glumly and stare down at your plate.

'You seem a little flat,' your mother says. 'Oui, oui,' you say. She looks at you oddly.

'What about going back on antidepressants again? You've been off them for a while. Might help?'

You sigh. By the time you hit 19, everyone in your family was on antidepressants and in intensive counselling—everyone but the dog and your father, who seemed to be the source of the problem.

'I think it's pretty normal to be depressed after two years travelling the world.' You think of the stillness of suburbia, of living with families, and how it just makes people sick.

'Well, what about seeing that psychologist your stepfather sees? She's very good. He's not isolating as much, seems to be making real progress.' She puts her hand on your shoulder, stands up. 'I'll go get her business card, alright?'

'Uh-huh.' As you wait for your mother to return you try and think of what Jacqueline would say. You're pretty sure she'd toss her glossy hair over one shoulder and mutter baise toi.

Your mother rings you after Christmas. You talk about Helen Garner's new book and the latest mass shooting in the U.S. and your stepfather's progress with a new therapist. Then naturally the conver- sation turns to Gerry.

'I think he has some transference issues,' she says.

'Right,' you say. You start doodling on a pad, drawing a person's brain, turning it into a dark storm cloud. 'Why's that?'

'Well, every time the school bell rings across the road he starts to bark.'

'Perhaps he's just alarmed by bells. Dogs don't like high frequen- cies.'

'Maybe. But I think there's more to it. I think he heard a bell when he was performing in the dog shows as a puppy and now every time he hears it he associates it with stress.'

'Right,' you say. 'Like Pavlov's dog.'

'Exactly,' she says. 'It's classic transference stuff, don't you think?' You're pretty sure your mother doesn't even know what transference is.

'Sure. Well, you'd know.' You start to draw a dog with big bared teeth and a piece of cheese wedged in its ass like a wine cork, looking like it's going to explode.

When you hang up, you think of all the time on your mother's hands. Her ailing health. Archie's neuroses and Gerry's anxiety. The story of Pavlov's fucking dog. But mainly you think about the lottery of mental illness—that seems to affect dachshunds and daughters—and entire families in equal measure.

You think about your mother's need to control and discipline Gerry and your need to control her in narrative. Twisting and contorting her worst traits for a story, wringing her out like a rag for dramatic effect. Making the prose tight, the dialogue contained so you can recreate a version of her, lay her down on the page—somehow hold her there forever. Sit. Stay. Good dog! Cleverly writing her into a story where you are the wise and witty narrator and she the needy, neurotic one, rambling on and on down the phone.

Thinking about all this makes you feel suddenly tired. Over- whelmed. Perhaps you're a little anxious or depressed? Thinking about your mother and the dachshunds and yourself is a complete headfuck. Perhaps you should take yourself out for a walk? Or make yourself a soothing cup of tea? You're not really sure what to do so you flick on the kettle. And, as you wait for it to boil, you pace up and down the kitchen floor—lap after lap after lap—until your finally wear yourself out.

Grey Gum

Stephanie Holm

The grey gum in Mo's yard was a beacon in our neighbourhood. Its branches curled above the rooftops – above the old telegraph poles – and when we'd first moved to town and got lost exploring the streets, we'd looked for its leaves against the skyline and found our way home. It was the largest tree I'd ever seen; I couldn't reach around its base. Even when Lee joined me and we both stretched our arms around the trunk our fingers didn't touch.

The tree gave us shade and the cockatoos loved it but Old Ted, who lived in number 5, on the other side of Mo, said their unearthly screeching wrought his nerves. But a lot of things wrought Old Ted's nerves, from the apricot colour Mo had recently painted his house, to the noise of us kids or 'that blasted tree'.

He complained regularly to Mo. 'Inconsiderate the way that tree drops its leaves on my roof and blocks my gutters. You should do something about it.'

Mo shrugged, 'Humans shed hair, dogs shed fur, trees shed leaves. It's natural process. I do not do anything about it.' And he closed the gate in Old Ted's face, turned to me and winked. 'He old codger, yes?'

I nodded, giggling. 'Yes.'

'Look.' Mo bent and picked something from the grass. He held it out. 'First flower.'

It looked soft and fluffy, nothing like the roses and pansies in Mrs Brown's front garden. She lived across the road from us and always made me stop to admire her flowers. 'Constant care and chicken poo' was her stinking motto.

'But where are its petals?' I said as Mo dropped the flower into my hand.

Mo shrugged again. 'No petals?' I shrugged too. 'I guess so.'

I didn't take much notice of the tree over the next couple of weeks; I had other stuff to see to – until the big wind came. I walked out the morning after the big wind to find the ground covered in snow. Only, when I looked more closely, it wasn't snow but fallen blossoms from the grey gum. Our yard, Mo's yard and Old Ted's roof were all coated in creamy white flower fluff. The street smelled of honey.

My brother, Lee, sniffed the air

'It's the blossoms from Mo's tree,' I explained.

'You're making it up,' he said, in that superior way older siblings do.

'It's true.' I picked up a flower, which fell apart in my hand, 'Here, smell this.'

He leaned forward, sniffed and sneezed. 'It's better than chicken poo, anyway.' And that was as much of an acknowledgement and apology as you could expect from him.

'Oh no. Old Ted. Don't look,' Lee warned. 'Too late, he's coming.

You had to look, didn't you?' 'I couldn't help it,' I said.

Old Ted huffed and grumbled his way over to us. He looked at the remains of the gum flower I held. 'You watch, it'll attract the foxes next.'

'What will?'

'Those flowers, and speaking of flowers—'

'C'mon.' Lee grabbed my arm. 'Sorry Ted, gotta go, or else we'll miss the bus.' And Lee made me run, even though the morning was already sweltering.

We rounded the corner.

'What foxes? Foxes don't eat flowers,' I puffed. Lee shook his head. 'He just likes to complain.'

It wasn't until later that night that we understood Old Ted's words about the foxes. Gran thought there was an intruder in the yard. She woke Mum, who woke Dad, who tripped on a stray slipper, which woke me. I thumped my fist on the bunk above.

'Lee,' I hissed. 'Something's going on.'

I followed the sound of Dad rattling 'round in the kitchen draws, then the torch beam that flicked on.

Lee yawned behind me but it turned to a gasp as we heard the noises that had disturbed Gran: a high-pitched screeching and chat- tering outside the back door. I don't know how we'd slept through it.

'What is it?' I whispered, trying to keep my voice from trembling.

The noises didn't sound human.

Dad unlocked the door.

'Dad, I don't think you should go out there.' But he did.

We pressed our noses against the flyscreen as Dad shone the torch about. Something flapped above his head and I ducked. He flicked the torch beam up. It lit up the grey gum trunk in Mo's yard.

Eyes shone back at us. 'It's ok, kids.'

There was a protesting screech and a whooshing as something flapped away from the light.

'Really?' Lee squeaked. I shuffled out behind him. In the torch- light, a grey-headed, orange-bodied bat hung upside down, its nose buried in a cluster of blossoms.

That's how we discovered the foxes—the flying foxes.

For nights afterward, we used to sneak out to the yard after Mum and Dad and Gran had gone to bed. We'd take torches and spotlight, watching the flying foxes feast and fight in the grey gum. The foxes didn't seem to mind us watching. If anything, they were noisier.

Sometimes we saw other animals too. Smaller bats that fluttered just outside the torch beam. And once, something scurrying up the trunk.

'A mouse?' I asked Lee.

We watched it for a while as it licked sap from the trunk, then it must have got tired of being in the spotlight and launched itself off the tree. But it didn't fall. It sort of parachuted over Mo's back fence.

'That mouse just flew!'

Lee shook his head. 'It wasn't a mouse, it was a glider,' he said as he climbed down from the veranda roof.

I stayed, hoping to spot the glider again—until Lee made me go inside.

'I hope it comes back tomorrow. I want to see it again.'

But the next evening was hot and humid

Gran sniffed the air before saying goodnight. 'Storm's brewing,' she said. 'Should be a doozy. Goodnight you two.'

'Goodnight Gran,' we chorused, but after the light had gone off in Gran's room we climbed back on to the veranda roof. The corrugat- ed iron was still warm on our backsides and, as we sat there, clouds drifted in. The sky started grumbling. There were flashes, white, far off—the beginnings of a storm. We watched as the lightning moved, now flickering all around. Then the thunder rumbled in. I tugged Lee's arm. 'We should get—'

A bolt of lightning shot down. It hit the grey gum. The light flared, engulfing the tree and vanished. The crack-boom that followed shook us, shook the roof, shook the whole street. Lights flicked on in windows. We leapt off the veranda, down the drainpipe and ducked under cover just as the rain started.

The grey gum smoked, but it was still standing. The air smelt wet, tangy, and left a metallic taste in our mouths. I blinked and it was as if the lightning struck again, imprinted on my eyeballs.

We waited and watched in case the tree burst into flame or decided to drop. Neither happened. The rain continued to fall—heavier now— and the lights in the neighbour's windows slowly blinked back out.

'You're shivering,' said Lee.

'You are too,' I replied, and my teeth continued to chatter, even after I laid in bed and pulled the blankets over my head.

The next morning Lee and I woke later than usual. Sun streamed around the curtain edges and we could hear voices outside, includ- ing Old Ted's. Lee was for staying in bed but I went to see what was happening. It seemed as if the whole street had congregated in Mo's backyard, looking up at the grand old gum. I stayed in our yard and watched them through a gap in the fence.

Even Gran was over there, pottering around behind the group. She disappeared behind the tree trunk. A minute later she reappeared. There was something stiff hanging from her hand. The others turned to her.

Old Ted stopped mid-sentence to stare. 'What is it?' 'Flying fox.'

Old Ted nodded, as if the dead bat proved his point. 'It'll die, you know.' He thumped the bark and repeated his words. 'It'll die.'

'Perhaps.' Mo stretched his arms wide. It looked as if he was going to say something more, but then his arms dropped and, 'I keep it,' is all he said.

This seemed to end the conversation. The others muttered, shook their heads and wandered back to their houses.

Gran passed Mo the dead bat. 'You keep it,' she offered.

As summer drifted into autumn we watched the leaves on the grey gum turn brown and drop.

One Friday afternoon, a particularly gusty wind tore the last leaves from their branches and deposited them on Old Ted's roof.

We were playing in the leaf litter when Old Ted stomped across. 'I saw those leaves fall into my gutter.'

Mo straightened from the herb garden he'd been working in and pointed up.

'No more leaves, no more fall in gutter.' And then he smiled, which made Old Ted crankier.

Old Ted stomped away and returned with some neighbours he'd managed to round up. He pointed to the tree. 'It's a danger to the neighbourhood,' he began, and glared at those he'd mustered. Mrs Brown cleared her throat, making a noise like a squeaky door, and in an equally squeaky voice said, 'Unsightly.'

Old Ted nodded but nobody else spoke up, so, he continued.

'A hazard—the next big wind will bring it down.' Still none of the others spoke, so, Old Ted was forced to sum up. 'And if it falls on my property you're footing the bill.'

But the next big wind didn't bring it down and they were still arguing come Spring. The tree was still standing, though its branches were bare, its bark had faded and Mo hadn't been invited to the annual community potluck dinner—so Lee and I escaped the dinner early to take him a plate of food.

'Thanks big much,' he said. We sat beside him as he finished Mum's potato bake.

'Tree not dead,' he said, suddenly, pointing with a forkful of Mrs Brown's casserole.

I looked at the tree but the only life I saw was a pair of sulphur-crested cockatoos. One was half-hidden in a hollow high amongst the dead branches. I watched the pair, trying to work out what Mo meant until—

'Pah!' He spat out a mouthful of mushed casserole. 'Disgusting,' he explained.

Later that night, Lee and I sat on the veranda roof once more and shone the torch on the grey gum. I don't think we really expected to see anything but Mo's words had made us curious.

'Look.' I made Lee hold the light still. A pair of eyes flashed.

There was something else alive in the tree.

After a time, the owner of the eyes grew brave and a brush- tail possum darted out of the hollow it had been hiding in. It ran down the trunk and leapt on to Mo's compost where it sat eating the remains of Mrs Brown's casserole.

I thought I began to see what Mo meant. So, I kept an eye on that tree. I saw the possum most evenings and watched the cockatoos fly back and forth, in and out of their hollow most days.

Just before Christmas an unusually loud chorus of screeching burst from Mo's yard. The two cockatoos were up in the tree but as I watched another, smaller cockatoo poked its crest out of the hollow. It looked about before jumping onto the branch beside its parents. Another crest took its place. Soon three young cockatoos perched, screeching beside their screeching parents.

I laughed. Old Ted donned earmuffs. He wore them all summer.

Gyne

Edyn Carter

My Grand Ant has humongous feelers, six spindly legs and a huge, bulbous bottom. With my eyes shut so tightly that rainbows burst under my eyelids; that is how I imagine her. I'm flopped out flat on the porch wearing my best Spring dress to impress the Grand Ant. A warm breeze tickles my cheeks. I imagine thousands of tiny ants that look just like her are marching out of my nostrils and across my face. My Grand Ant is the size of a house. She has to be, I think. How else would she have had room for all of her children? Grand Ant, I decide, has ten eyes; one for each child she had to watch.

Mamma told me to wait here for the Grand Ant. I've been lying out here all day. Since Mamma's belly grew, she's tired; but she wasn't always. I remember Mamma pushing me on our swing. She'd push me so high that I felt like I was in space. I hope my Grand Ant will push me on the swing. Mamma's asleep now and I'm angry that the Grand Ant will wake her when she arrives. She'd better not wake Mamma with her pincers, I decide, or I'll have to squish her with my shoe! My Grand Ant has two mighty pincers and she needs to keep them away from my Mamma, I think.

I'm startled out of my daydream by a car and noise in the gravel. There's a crunching of rocks, followed by lazy dragging of feet; the Grand Ant. When I see her, I'm disappointed. She doesn't have feelers. Her bottom's bulbous and her legs are spindly but there are only two of them. The rest of her is spindly too. I think she looks more like a Grand Spider than an ant. Her face is pointy with small black eyes that match her shiny hair. She shuffles toward me. I notice that her skin matches her old suitcase and how her arms and legs move like they are all separate. Grand Ant is just like a spider, indeed. 'Hello, Grand Ant!' She looks at me curiously, pushing her nose and her eyebrows close together. She looks down at my legs, giving them a short nod.

'Close your legs, girl. What if the neighbour boys saw you?' I don't understand what the boys would think if they did see me. She doesn't bother to explain. I keep my legs as they are.

I'm pushing myself on our swing. The warm air crashes over my body as I sail upward and dive back into it. Suddenly there is someone in front of me, too close as I rocket back down to Earth. To keep from crashing into her, I dig my toes into the dirt, forcing myself to stop.

It's the Grand Ant. She says she's brought me a present and is waving me off the swing and inside.

She shoves it toward me; my first doll, wrapped in crumpled pink paper. It's an old thing with a hard body, orange hair and one eye that only half blinks. Its hair has been cut short on one side and its curls are more like knots. It's wearing a soft green dress, like mine. When I run my fingers over it, one of its tiny pearl buttons falls off. Grand Ant tells me, proudly, that it was Mamma's when she was a little girl 'like me'. Mamma sighs dramatically and tells me that she remembers taking care of 'her' as though she were real. I smile and nod at them both, holding the doll by its hair. Grand Ant clicks her tongue at me and forces my arms into a stiff cradle.

'There,' she says. 'You'll make a fine mother one day; that's what I expect.'

'Thank you, Grand Ant,' I say, and I mean it. I think that, perhaps, Grand Ant isn't as bad with kids as Mamma tells Father she is while Grand Ant's not around to hear her.

I say that my arms ache. Grand Ant laughs. 'That's how a mother's arms are supposed to feel.'

In the kitchen that evening, I hear harsh whispering that is not my Mamma's and then there is silence. After a moment, Mamma appears. She speaks to me in a low voice, her eyes flicking from the kitchen to me.

'Please, call Grand Ant 'Grandmother', or 'Antonia', from now on,' she says.

I nod but I'm only half listening. Instead, I'm seeing. I see Mamma. With her huge round stomach and her thin limbs I think she must be an ant like the Grand Ant. I wonder, then, if I'm also an ant or if I'll be an ant one day with a stomach that round. I imagine it like a growth; a great swollen thing which has made Mamma more pimple than person. I imagine what would be inside if it burst open. I like my stomach as it is, I decide.

Three nights later, I'm sitting on my bedroom floor, brushing my doll's hair before bed. I brush it too hard and it tears out in clumps. I think she's beautiful even without most of her hair. I tell her she's pretty, smooth her dress until it's straight again and kiss her nose. I love my doll. I decide I should name her because that's what mothers do. 'Winona. That's your name.'

I notice a spider on the ceiling. It's black and rounder than any spider I've seen before. It reminds me of Mamma. I stand up, shakily, on my bed to peer at it. Inches from my face, I decide to blow on it to scare it away. When I do, the spider falls apart. It is a thousand baby spiders. They scatter across my wall and I scream.

That night I wake to hear Mamma screaming, too. My Grand Ant orders me back to my room. With my door cracked open, I see Mamma crying in the reflection of the bathroom mirror across the hall. Her eyes are so red, and in the yellow light she looks sick. I feel sick, too. Father runs from the bedroom to see what's wrong, though his eyes are half closed from being woken up. When my Father and my Grand Ant walk her out the door and into the car, she walks blood into the hallway by my door. After Mamma's gone, I wet a rag and try to clean the blood from the carpet. The blood spreads. In the end it stains pink, twice the size it had been.

Mamma returns the next evening. The night is warm, but in my house the air is silent and cold. Mamma's face looks grey. My Grand Ant coughs from her chair and it seems to bounce off the walls, ringing in my ears. I try to show Mamma what's left of Winona's hair, but she only stares at her. When they think I'm asleep that night, my door creaks open and I hear the shuffling of Grand Ant's feet. In the morning, Winona is gone from my room. I find her two days later in the garbage can outside, and I dig her out but she is too broken to fix.

At thirteen years old, I hear Mamma laugh again. She squeals, and I rush into the bathroom to see what's wrong. She turns from the mirror to me and I see the way the yellow light makes her blonde curls shine and her cheeks look rosy. She laughs and then cries. We sit at the dinner table and I smile because she's happy. I guess I'm supposed to be happy, too, though I don't understand why. She doesn't explain because it doesn't cross her mind that she'd need to. My parents chatter about names. They talk quickly and with their mouths full. Remembering my doll, I tell them that they should call it Winona, if it's a girl.

'Oh, Winona's an old person's name. You can call your own daughter Winona one day, if you like it so much.' The way Mamma talks about my future daughter is certain. I just nod and then I'm quiet.

Not quite nine months later, my Father, Mamma, Grand Ant and I are running to the car. The hospital is too bright. The waiting room stinks like Grand Ant's hair dye. The hallways are too empty. Grand Ant takes a Bible from her purse and reads it to me. She asks if I know any scripture. When I say no, she begins to tell me about the Virgin Mary. I don't understand how her story can be true because I know how babies are made but I take her word for it because it's not ladylike to argue.

'Virginity is the most important thing a woman should keep if she respects herself,' whispers Grand Ant. I'm suddenly embarrassed, because I suppose I should be, so I look away and laugh. Grand Ant is silent after this.

I close my eyes and imagine I am Mamma. I hear the beeping of machines. I imagine doctors groping me with plastic gloves. I remember Mamma's stomach that night with Grand Ant and imagine my stomach is round. Suddenly, it's getting fatter, popping the buttons on my blouse. It's getting so round that it spills out over the top of my skirt. I watch it grow with purple veins like snakes under my skin.

I swell and swell until I'm tremendous and round, my belly button popping outward. I think about myself beginning to grow feelers. They sprout from my head and grow large. I imagine myself growing four extra legs, short and skinny. I'm an ant; the Grand Ant. I'm an ant and my belly is big. It's so big that my body can no longer hold what is inside. My stomach is so large that it pops. But there are no smiling babies inside me. Instead, I imagine myself bursting and thousands of tiny black spiders erupt from my growth. They scuttle out in a mass and smother me. I am growing again; my feelers replaced by two more legs, my ant legs getting longer, arching at the knees as they hit the floor. The spiders cover my skin and drop to the floor as I expand. When I finish growing, I am no longer an ant. I am a spider.

When I wake, my Grand Ant is asleep next to me. Mamma screams in her room down the hall. A baby cries, making my skin itch.

I feel him looking at me. Thinking he's upset me, he reaches over and gently squeezes my hand. 'Did you hear me?'

I'd heard him but in the same moment something had caught my eye. He follows my gaze to the large black spider in the corner of the ceiling. Quietly, I slip out of bed, picking up a heel from the shoe-rack. In one swing I hit the spider, watching as it flattens to a mark on the wall.

'Did you know that some female spiders eat their young?' The question sounds more like a fact. He doesn't respond. I feel his confu- sion as he watches me. Grand Ant was always more spider than ant.

'Hello? Did you hear me?' He doesn't pay attention to my question. 'Hmm?' I turn to him, catching his hopeful, urging look.

'Do you think that, maybe, it's time for us to start thinking about having kids? We've been married a few months now.' He smiles at me.

My silence hangs too long. 'Yeah,' I say after a minute and I force a smile.

He moves to kiss me. I say that I'm happy. I say that I love him. I ask why I wouldn't want to have his children, of course. I say that I've always wanted to have children. I say it because there's no way to say that I, too, am more spider than I could ever be an ant.

Socks

Rhona Hammond

It was about seven o'clock on Sunday night when the phone rang. I was in the middle of folding the washing and the girls were building something in Lego. It was Jenny, their stepmother. My ex's new wife. The one he left me for. I have to deal with her so I just do. But it would be good if she wasn't in my life.

'Hi Jenny. What's up?'

'Oh, nothing much, I was just wondering if, er, maybe you were a bit short on school socks? Because we seem to have a lot of them over here. Maybe I could send some over?'

Weird. Why the hell was she calling me about socks? I mean, just shove some in their bags. But, as I looked at the piles of laundry on the kitchen bench: theirs, mine, I realised that there was a sock shortage going on and so I decided to take it as the friendly, helpful gesture that it appeared to be.

'Thanks, yes, I think we do need some socks.'

There was an awkward pause because I couldn't think of a good way to end the call. I didn't want to say 'was there anything else?' because I didn't want anything else. I wanted her out of my house. Off my phone.

'Look, this is really inappropriate so, you know, just tell me, but I wanted to talk to you about Michael. It's just that we're going through a rough patch at the moment and I don't know what to do.'

I think I was a bit stunned and I think I panicked. I didn't want the girls hearing this call so I sprinted for the kitchen and then out onto the balcony. And she was talking while I did that but I wasn't listening.

'Em, right. Look, Jenny, I just don't think that '

'I know, I know, but he doesn't want me to speak to my family or, well, anyone really.'

'Uhuh.'

'He's never here and I'm left alone with the kids, sometimes all of them, and he isn't listening. He says I just nag him all the time and I can never find anything when he asks me and that it's all my fault but I have no idea where his black jeans are, I don't think I've washed them in weeks.'

Those jeans are probably at the new girlfriend's house. Scrunched up on a floor somewhere. And he'll be telling her about how cold and nagging his wife is and how she doesn't understand him and, Jesus, I hope he's had the snip because if he fathers any more kids I'll . . . I'll do what, exactly? None of this is my problem. Except that it is.

'I just really wanted to ask you, since you separated, have you found peace? Are you free?'

Have I found peace. Am I free.

'Absolutely. Thank God I'm free. Free of him and his bullshit. It's great. I have this amazing mindfulness calendar and I change the message every day.'

Except, of course, I didn't actually say that. I didn't want to be rude to the woman who had been shagging my husband behind my back for months, while I was pregnant and giving birth and staying home with my second child. If her ex hadn't called me and told me what they were up to I might never have known. Instead I said, 'Yes. I'm happy.'

Am I at peace. Am I free. No. I am not. I pretend I am but I am actually sick with anger at the pair of them with their twin girls and their fancy wedding. I try not to get angry about the fact that I'm living here in this tiny apartment while they have a new house that he swore he couldn't afford when we were divorcing. There is no point getting angry about it, even though I found the banking records that showed how he took money out of our account for over a year before he left. I could never understand why he was always short of cash but it was going into his war chest. I can't get angry about that because I need all my energy for my girls and my job.

I suddenly thought about her kids and who was watching them right now while she was dumping this on me so I said,

'Where are Jacqueline and Freida?'

'Oh, Fred's asleep and Jacq's watching TV.'

And that made me even angrier because it drives me nuts the way she just parks my girls in front of a screen every chance she gets and then they come home after a weekend at their place and they are all wired because they haven't burned off any energy because they aren't allowed outside because they might have to be supervised and they might get dirty and Jesus Christ. It's exhausting.

'Mum?'

'Jenny, that's one of the girls calling me. I'd better go. I, erm, well I hope things are. I. Hmm. Well, yes. I'll see you soon.' I think she said something but I am not sure what and then I hung up and went back into the kitchen.

'Who was on the phone?' asked Olivia, nosy for signs of a new boyfriend.

'It was just Jenny.'

'Oh. Daddy says she's really stupid.'

The Guide hall always looks so spooky amongst the trees. One big old spotlight on the building has to secure the whole muddy car park. The girls haven't been to Guides for a while because I've been working late and it's too much to expect Mum to take them and collect them. She does enough for me. I applied the hand brake and took a moment, breathing and slouching, gathering myself together. I cricked my neck and rubbed my eyes.

That's when I saw it. Michael's car. Why? Oh God, is he shagging one of the other mothers? I joined a few other parents arriving at the concrete steps outside the door of the hall. The girls came flooding out, about twenty of them, and I gave the car key to Suzy, told Olivia to hop in the front.

'Daddy came tonight! He's talking to Brown Owl.'

'Ok. You guys hop into the car, I'll be there in a minute.'

I didn't get as far as the door. I heard him before I saw him.

'. . . so she hasn't brought them for a few weeks, eh? She can be unreliable, my ex, tends to run a bit hot and cold, you know. How are the girls coping?'

Brown Owl made no reply. She's a tough old bird, chief librar- ian at the high school. I imagined her standing there in the empty wooden hall with Michael, just holding her peace, watching and judging.

I wasn't in the mood for Michael and his bullshit. I turned and ducked back to the car.

'Did Daddy say why he came along tonight?' I asked the girls. 'Yes, he brought some socks for us. We left them at his house.'

Olivia waved a plastic bag. 'Right. Anything else?'

Heads shook. I started the car and drove home. I saw his silhou- ette in the rearview mirror and shuddered.

When the girls were in bed and my tea had gone cold I found the bag of socks on the sofa. I untied the knot, shook them onto the coffee table and started to pair them up because, of course, she hadn't bothered to do that. There was a note on a piece of fancy writing paper. The message said, 'Leah, I need some help. I don't know what to do. Jenny.'

I sat back on the sofa and stared at it for a while. I considered tearing it up and ignoring it. Had I found peace? No. Would letting the other woman go to the wall bring me peace?

No. I made another cup of tea and did some stretches for my back and neck.

I stuck a pair of socks back into the plastic bag with the piece of paper. On the reverse I wrote the name and number of my solicitor. I tied the bag closed again. I would tell Olivia that Jenny had accidentally included some socks I didn't recognise. They could take them back this weekend.

Michael got a house in the divorce but I kept his mother, Rachel. When she refused to wholeheartedly embrace his change of partner, when she dared to suggest he was behaving like a fool towards me, he had cut her off. He said she was disloyal, that she didn't love him enough but she just shrugged and told him to grow up.

Rachel picked the girls up from school on Thursdays and was waiting with dinner when I got home. That Thursday night she had opened a bottle of wine and poured me a glass. I went to the girls' room to give them a kiss and then came back to sit at the kitchen bench.

‘Oh, should have asked them to set the table,’ I said and went to get up again but Rachel stopped me and jerked her head in a ‘got some- thing to tell you’ manner. Quick before the girls come.

‘I ran into Jenny at the supermarket today. She wouldn’t let me get away. Going on about things being difficult with Michael and could I help her, did I have any advice. She held onto my arm, I had to ask her to let go! And then, and this is the bit that makes me furious, she starts to tell me about Suzy and Olivia and how badly behaved they are at her house and how you feed them rubbish and that’s a big part of the problem! I said, Jenny, I said, I know my grand-daughters very well and they are angels and Leah feeds them a healthy, varied diet and I don’t know what you’re talking about.’

I drank my wine and shook my head. ‘I’m sorry Rachel. I’m sorry it’s like this.’

‘Don’t be love, it’s all his fault. He created this mess.’

After Rachel left, when the girls were in bed and the dishes done, I retrieved the bag of socks. I threw the note out, put the socks away and recycled the plastic bag.

Arranged Marriage

Sanchana Venkatesh

38 / 6ft / Hindu Tamil Brahmin/ Masters / $100,000 p.a. / Upper middle-class family / Handsome groom from Sydney / Seeks fair- skinned, good looking, educated Hindu Tamil Brahmin girl / 18 to 32 / 5'2 to 5'9 / No dowry

'This is the person they want you to meet?' asked Paula, rolling her eyes. 'I can't believe people post ads in the classifieds when we have Tinder or RSVP these days.'

Nithya laughed, her brown eyes crinkling. 'You know I haven't had much luck online. I'm meeting him to make my mum and dad happy. It's not like I'm agreeing to marry him at first sight.'

They re-read the advertisement in the Indian Chronicle out loud and burst into laughter again.

'I better head off,' said Nithya. 'I've got to turn myself into a fair and good-looking Indian bride and that doesn't happen in an hour.' She hugged her best friend, paid for her breakfast and walked towards her parked car.

Humming to the beats of Rhianna, Nithya wondered once again why she had agreed to see this man. She hadn't been lying to Paula when she'd mentioned not having much luck with online dating or that she was trying to make her parents happy. But if she was being completely honest, her parents hadn't given her much of a choice. They had talked about how they were not getting any younger and yearning to go back to India, but also wanting to see her "settle down" before they did that. It didn't matter she was a senior account manager in a PR firm or had her unit in Lane Cove. She had finally agreed to meet some men of their choice and Mr Classified's guy was the first they'd picked.

Nithya parked near the kerb in front of her parents' single-lev- el red brick house. It was the same home she'd grown up in and her room, with its Green Day and Linkin Park posters, remained untouched. Each time she visited, she transformed into the fourteen year old, filled with teenage angst. She rang the doorbell and waited, listening to the hum of the neighbour's lawn mower on a Sunday morning. Her mother, Saroj, opened the door and greeted her with a hug and an appraising look. 'Time to get you out of those jeans and into a sari.'

'Lovely to see you too, Ma,' replied Nithya, following her mother into the house. The scent of chillies and peppers tickled her nose as she walked into the kitchen, sending her into fits of sneezes. Through sniffles, she asked, 'What's happening here?' The kitchen was laden with food—plates of samosas, potato bhajiyas, and other food she didn't recognise. 'What's all this?'

'Oh, just a little food to welcome Arjun and his family,' said her mother. 'It's the right thing to do.'

'Isn't it just him and his parents?' asked Nithya. 'It looks like you have enough here to feed everyone from India.'

'This is why you are still single in your thirties. You don't know how to win a man's heart. Back in my day . . . '

'Ugh, Ma. I'm going to get dressed.' Nithya walked out of the kitchen, sampling a bhajiya on the way to her room. Her mother's voice rang behind her with warnings about watching her weight and not getting her oily fingers on the sari. Wiping her hands on her jeans, she entered the room and saw a pastel pink chiffon sari with little diaman- tes on her bed. She felt the soft, papery texture between her fingers and grimaced at the thought of looking like fairy floss ready to be pulled apart and devoured.

'Ma,' she called out.

'Yes, you have to wear it,' yelled back her mother.

Nithya cursed herself for agreeing to this meeting. She hated being paraded around like an item for sale. If it had been up to her, she and this guy would have met for a coffee or over a drink. But her parents would not hear of it. They'd jumped the second she had hesitantly agreed to meet this man and had called the number on the ad. Her parents and his had spoken like long-lost friends. Before she knew it, a meeting had been set without a word being exchanged between her and this man.

Saroj walked in and offered to help. Nithya rarely wore saris and the few times she did, her mother had helped her drape it, deftly making the pleats and tucking them into the petticoat around her waist. This time, as her mother wrapped the sari around her, Nithya felt it stran- gling her, trapping the woman inside.

'This is so not me,' said Nithya making a face as her mother put two gold bangles on each of her wrists and dotted her forehead with a bindi. She allowed her mother to braid her hair, leaving loose curls on the sides. She made up her face with a bit of eyeliner and a dab of lipstick.

'I wish you wouldn't go out in the sun so much,' muttered her mother, offering Nithya some foundation which she refused. 'It makes your skin so dark.' Before Nithya could retort, the doorbell rang. She heard her father open the door while her mother trotted out to welcome the visitors.

Nithya looked at her bedroom window and wondered for a moment if she should just give the whole thing a miss. She heard voices—mumbles that were foreign to her, her mother's high-pitched voice when she got excited, and her father's dulcet tones. Instead of jumping out the window, she took a deep breath and walked out to greet the visitors with her head held high. She found it awkward walking in her sari and wished her mother hadn't been so fussed about the outfit.

She listened as her parents ushered Arjun and his family into the living room. 'The traffic is getting worse each year,' she heard his mother say in her thick Indian accent. She waited until they were seated and then waltzed in, with a smile plastered on her face.

'Hello,' she said, while simultaneously tripping on her sari. 'Whoops!' She gave a wry smile, pointed to her sari and said, 'Not used to this thing.' The stony look from Arjun's mother wiped the smile off her face.

Her own mother hastily introduced her. 'This is Nithya. She's a senior account manager at Wilson-Brown. She's been there for five years.' There was a hint of pride in her mother's voice and Nithya's eyes pricked. No matter how often her mother told her she should have studied medicine, she was proud of what Nithya had accomplished in her career. Arjun's family however, did not seem impressed. 'You work long hours?' was his mother's way of introducing herself.

'Sometimes,' nodded Nithya. 'And you are . . . ?' She held out her right hand to his mother.

Arjun's parents looked affronted. His mother recovered first and held her palms together, leaving Nithya's hand dangling mid-air. Her mother jumped in with the introductions.

'Mr and Mrs Krishnan, and Arjun,' she said, pointing to each of them in turn. Nithya nodded at them and finally turned to check out Arjun. She usually stayed away from Indian men but could see he was okay-looking. Not handsome, but not bad either. He was dark- skinned with gelled hair and piercing brown eyes. He sported a slight moustache and she made a mental note to tell him he'd be better off without it. He was dressed in jeans and a grey collared shirt. He smiled when introduced and Nithya, noticing his yellowed teeth, cringed while smiling back.

'Nithya, why don't you take Arjun to the backyard? I'll bring some tea and snacks out for you,' said her mother, giving Nithya permission to escape the glowering looks of Mrs Krishnan. As he rose to follow her, she realised he wasn't six feet tall. Being around five feet, five inches herself, she didn't have to crane her neck too far to meet his gaze. Out in the backyard, Nithya felt her shoulders drop as she let out a deep breath she hadn't realised she was holding. Arjun stood with his hands in his pockets, watching two ibises on the fence fight for food.

Nithya tried to lighten the mood. 'This is weird. I've never done one of these arranged meetings before.'

'Oh, really?' asked Arjun, raising his eyebrows. 'I've done more than I can count on both hands.'

It was Nithya's turn to raise her eyebrows. 'And you still haven't found someone suitable?'

He gave a wry smile and didn't reply. Nithya continued. 'What do you do for work?'

'I work in finance. For Westpac.' 'Do you enjoy it?'

He shrugged. 'It's a job. Why? Do you enjoy yours?'

'Of course! I love mine. Sure, there are days when I want to pull my hair out but, generally, I love it. Wouldn't be doing it otherwise.'

He nodded slowly. 'Do you plan on continuing to work after marriage?'

Nithya laughed then straightened her face. 'You're serious? Yes, I plan on working till my retirement.'

'What about when you have children?'

The clouds above covered the sun, creating a shadow over the backyard and making it seem smaller than before.

'I'm still undecided on the children-front,' said Nithya. 'But even if I do have kids, I plan on returning to work after maternity leave. My mum worked while I was growing up—it's good for kids to see both parents working anyway.'

Arjun let out a long 'hmmm.'

'Didn't your mum work?' asked Nithya. He shook his head.

Nithya bit back a retort, marvelling at her self-restraint. 'What do you enjoy doing? Any hobbies?'

Arjun took a while to think about this. 'I guess I enjoy watching sport on telly, playing board games.'

'Nothing outdoors?' asked Nithya.

'Nah, I'm not much of an outdoorsy person.'

Nithya's jaw dropped. He was the first guy she'd met in all her years who wasn't outdoorsy. 'Well, I love the beach, running, cycling, and playing sport,' she said.

'Is that why you're so dark?' he asked.

'Excuse me?' Nithya blinked. 'Did you just ask me if I was dark?

As in dark-skinned?'

He nodded. 'The ad clearly said "fair-skinned" and, let's face it, you're not.'

'No, I'm not,' said Nithya, feeling a burning sensation in her chest and clenching her fists. 'And I'm okay with that. But in case you haven't looked in a mirror, you're not fair-skinned either. In fact, compared to a lot of people in this country, neither of us is fair- skinned.'

'I am lighter than you. I want my children to be light-skinned. And who have a mother around to look after them and not out galli- vanting with colleagues.'

Nithya gritted her teeth and watched the smaller of the two ibises soar with its reward, leaving the bigger one hanging off the fence. Before she could gather her thoughts to form a coherent sentence, her mother appeared with a tray of food and two cups of tea.

'Some chai, Arjun? And pakoras?' She lay the tray on the table and held a cup out to him. Arjun reached over when Nithya inter- rupted. 'I don't think Arjun can stay for chai, Ma. He has to leave urgently.'

She turned to Arjun and smiled, 'Let me show you and your parents out.'

After walking an irate Mr and Mrs Krishnan out the house, Nithya headed back to her room and shut the door to tune out her mother's moans about her rude behaviour. She lay on her bed in her petticoat and blouse, staring at the posters of her adolescent heroes while the pink sari lay crumpled on the floor. Her phone buzzed, and she looked at the screen. It was a message from a guy named Eric on Tinder: I feel like we have a lot in common and that my mother would approve of you. Nithya burst out laughing and began typing her reply.

Red Dust & Pearls

Marlish Glorie

Nola couldn't stomach the poets. But I never thought she'd try and kill one. She was getting ahead of herself. It was one thing to badmouth the snotty-nosed twerps behind their backs, bumping one off in broad daylight though, was a whole different ball game. The first I heard about it all was when two policemen turned up on my front doorstep holding copies of a slim volume of poems titled Divinity.

It would seem that Nola while reversing her clapped-out bambino fiat from the car park of the writers' centre where she worked as a volunteer, had backed over not only a poet but a prize-winning one. The poets, of whom there were too many according to Nola, were outraged. They asserted that the mowing down of one-of-their-own had been premeditated and were busy penning poems they could perform as means of nonviolent protest. The poets had become, in literary parlance, performance poets. No matter the venue or that the audience was always branch stacked with other poets. Or this is what Nola told me, along with the fact that the poets ate their own body weight in food at every performance.

I decided, the policemen and I needed to sit down and have a talk, man to man. I invited them into my home where I told them to pull up a pew. I gave them mugs of tea and freshly baked damper with generous dollops of butter. I was buggered if those bumbling show ponies were going to paint Nola as some sort of criminal. So, while one of the now greasy-fingered policemen flicked through his copy of Divinity, I explained how Nola's life hadn't amounted to much, and how at the age of seventy she was finally starting to realize a lifetime's dream of writing a romance novel called Red Dust and Pearls. Both the policemen furrowed their brows and jutted out their bottom lips.

I put another chunk of damper onto each of their tin plates. Then I sat myself down to give them an outline of Nola's novel which is about a beautiful young woman named, Marigold, whose a pilot for the Royal Flying Doctor Service up North, in the outback. Being headstrong yet tenderhearted, she soon catches the fancy of a local cattle baron. Brock, the cattle baron, is ruggedly handsome and filthy rich. And when he's not zooming around in a helicopter, he's on a stock horse galloping across the dusty red plains with the wind raking his sun-bleached hair, a rollie dangling from the corner of his mouth. And at night, when the inky sky is ablaze with stars, he's sitting by the campfire, sharing a brew and a yarn with the stockmen, his loyal cattle dog, Bluey, lying asleep by his feet.

The policemen, while eating damper and sipping tea, nodded their appreciation.

'Sounds good,' said the policeman with the greasy fingers, who'd now fashioned his copy of Divinity into a cylindrical tube which he spied through. 'I wouldn't mind being Brock.'

For Nola, it was a far cry from her own life. She read romance novels by the truckload while cleaning houses and looking after her disabled adult son and knitting beanies for charity.

The prize-winning poet, who'd barely been touched by the rear bumper bar, according to Nola, had also wangled a paid residency at the writer's centre. Years earlier with the help of a fat grant she had written a couple of very slim volumes of poetry which were published. But Nola said that sales had been lousy, and the books ended up being pulped. The poet had a pen name—The Poetess, and her email address was poetess@ hotmail.com. She also had a stack of business cards made from recycled paper with Poetess for Hire printed on them. Nola thought the poetess was an oxygen thief. Who was I to argue?

Nola used to get real excited by her story and loved nothing more than telling me about the extra bits she'd tacked onto Red Dust & Pearls. She asked for my opinion whenever she saw me at the writers' centre, while we made cups of tea for the poets.Or mopped floors. Or took out the rubbish. Nola had made the mistake of going to the writing centre's A.G.M., where she'd put up her hand. Volunteering to do whatever was needed. I suppose it gave Nola the chance to discuss her work-in-progress with a gentleman like myself who appreciates the ways of a woman's heart.

'I'm having Brock rescue a Japanese tourist who's been taken by a six-metre crocodile. Then when the Royal Flying Doctor arrives to take the chewed-up and spat out tourist to Darwin Hospital, Brock meets Marigold, and sparks fly,' enthused Nola one day when we were cleaning the windows. 'What ya reckon?'

Clutching scrunched up newspaper and a bottle of Windex in my rubber-gloved hands, I gave her the thumbs up and told her I was stoked to be hanging out with a soon-to-be-famous writer. Nola's face crumpled and tears slid down her face. I put an arm around her shoul- ders and handed her my hanky.

I'm not sure how it all came about, the poetess wanting to read Nola's romance novel because her so-called feedback crushed poor Nola. You see while Nola was great at cooking up stories, her writing was a mess.

The poetess wore a pink nylon wig, and her website was a bragsite, carping on how she could do pretty well anything, including whistling Waltzing Matilda while doing backflips through burning hoops. But when she read Nola's romance novel, she whined how it was formulaic and sexist and would never get published.

Nola took it on the chin and muddled on with Red Dust & Pearls, putting commas where she thought they ought to go, looking up spelling in the dictionary, and shuffling paragraphs around until they were all roughly the same size. I helped by figuring out where Marigold should blush and when Brock should burn with desire.

Nola said, she'd only scratched the poetess with her car. The poets claimed she'd put her foot on the accelerator. Nola counter- claimed, she hadn't seen the poetess. The poets bellyached how they were a persecuted lot. And between them they supposedly had a gazillion photographs on their mobile phones as professed proof of the bambino fiat ploughing into their pin-up girl. The photographs which had been photo-shopped to look like the poetess had been backed over by a bulldozer repeatedly were posted on Instagram, Facebook and Twitter. In reality, she'd been boozing at a performance gig then stumbled dead drunk into the car park before crashing headfirst into Nola's car at the exact moment Nola was putting her key into the ignition.

Nola didn't mean to hit the poetess, although she might have been tempted. She told me about the day previous to the incident when she was washing dishes from yet another performance gig in the kitchen sink. The poetess, who was wearing a pink tee-shirt with the words—Vegan for the Voiceless—emblazoned on the front, trooped in and flung open the fridge door. She pointed to a block of cheese sitting on one of the shelves.

'This cheese is contaminating my food.'

Nola stared at the poetess and then at the cheese, wondering what was going on.

'Remove it,' said the poetess. 'Please,' she added sarcastically.

Nola dried her hands before picking up the cheese. 'I'll take it home.'

Ms Cheesed-off eyeballed Nola as if she was the hired help. She handed Nola one of her business cards before leaning back on the open fridge door. Nola glanced at the pink card with the words Love makes Poets printed on the front. To her horror, she heard herself say, 'Thanks.' By way of reply, the poetess gave a one-shouldered shrug

before leaving Nola to close the fridge door. It was at this point, Nola got stroppy. She was angry with herself for kowtowing to the woman.

Nola was adamant the poetess had merely sustained a graze to her forehead, and which had been put right with a couple of band-aids from the writing centre's first aid kit. The poets maintained that Nola's car was dented from having run over the poetess whose blood was now smudged onto the duco and soaked into the tread of the rear tyres. Pink nylon strands from her wig were found on the brake lights. The poets bleated how it was very nearly curtains for the poetess who was saved in the nick of time after being rushed to a nearby hospital. But due to complications would have on-going medical problems and a pronounced limp.

'I've been stitched-up,' lamented Nola, when I last saw her at the writer's centre.

I clicked my tongue.

The poets had managed, somehow, to fabricate an ironclad case against Nola. She ended up doing time in a rural minimum-securi- ty prison, where she continued to work on her novel. The first time I drove out to visit her, I was surprised to see her in such good spirits.

'I'm thinking,' Nola explained excitedly about her novel. 'When the noonday sun is high in a taut blue sky and baking the red earth, Brock and Marigold ought to go swimming in the cool, clear waters of a billa- bong where Brock hints to Marigold, he wants to marry her. What do you reckon?'

Reckon I could live with it, just fine.'

Each time I drove out to see Nola, her novel was getting closer to being finished. But then one day, she hit me with the news. 'The poetess, remember her? She's here now at the prison. She got a resi- dency.'

'Stone the crows.'

'I've stopped working on my novel.' 'Whoa! You're kidding me?'

'No. I think the poetess is right.' 'About what?'

'My novel, being sexist and predictable.'

'But it's my story,' I stammered. 'Don't cut me loose like this.' 'Them's the breaks.'

'What about Marigold?'

'Girl like her? She'll find another story.'

I stared down at my boots, noticing the red dust in its creases. Nola gave a weighty sigh. 'You should see her limp.'

I scratched my head. Nola was between a rock and a hard place. 'Me and the poetess have started a writer's group, Behind Bars

Performance Poets,' Nola explained carefully.' I went quiet.

'She thinks I'm gifted and shouldn't be wasting my time writing trash. We're writing an anthology of poetry together, Caged Dreams.'

My heart sank. Nola had written me off. She was on a roll. I was cactus.

Nola started to rabbit on about doing a poetry performance gig in the prison cafeteria and inviting the poets along.

The time had come for me to roll up my swag and shoot through. But I was gutted. I knew romance writers were a fickle two-faced lot, but to get knifed in the back like that? It had me beat. I never wanted to clap eyes on another romance writer ever again. Still, I put on a brave front and bid my fair-weather friend goodbye.

In the dying light of evening, I removed the rollie from behind my ear, lit it, and took a few drags. I started to walk out of the prison. My footsteps were heavy and slow as I made my way along an avenue of ghost gums. A bunch of pink and greys took off in flight. By the time I got to within cooee of the entrance, I'd finished my smoke and placed the butt into the top pocket of my checkered shirt. I stopped by the entrance where a kindly looking female guard stepped forward. She was holding my dog Bluey for me, on a leash. I tipped my hat. She gave me a smile before handing me back my most loyal friend.

Just One Night

Nicole Hodgson

It was just for one night. Helen could put up with anything for one night. She stretched the sheets tight across the guest bed, then smoothed out the quilt and plumped the pillows. Just one night. It echoed, around and around, like a mantra.

She hadn't heard from Pete since their mother's funeral three years earlier. She hadn't been sure where he was living at the time and she had no idea if her messages would reach him. But he had appeared at the chapel, like an unsettling wraith. Grey skin pock- marked with sores, dull sunken eyes, angry red marks on his hands from incessant scratching. She couldn't bring herself to hug him, let alone kiss him. She could only acknowledge their relationship, their once close bond, with a brief brush of his navy polyester sleeve. The suit hung from his bony shoulders and it reeked of op-shop. He asked to borrow money and she gave him fifty bucks. He had slipped away before the line of mourners had finished passing on their condolences.

Ever since that awful funeral she had expected a phone call. From a hospital or the police. Instead the voice on the phone had been Pete's. The husky tenor was still so familiar that it skewered her heart with a sharp remembrance of love. He must have been having a good day, because he sounded coherent and asked only to see her. She was so shocked to hear from him that she had blurted out an invitation to dinner and to stay the night. He said 'see you in a few days' then hung up before she could ask him anything. He was alive at least. Probably desperate for cash.

Helen folded and smoothed a fluffy towel, then laid it on the bed. She didn't bother with the sprig of rosemary or lavender that she would place on top for other guests, the friends that occasionally came to stay.

As she turned to leave the room, a framed poster caught her eye. The Triffids, playing at the Old Melbourne. May 1986. She had gone to that gig with Pete. He had bought that poster for her. Back when he actually had cash to spare. They had been so close in their twenties. Half a lifetime ago. They had shared friends, decrepit old mansions in Fremantle and Cottesloe, travels to India and Indone- sia. Everyone had loved him then, sharp, bold, restless Pete. He had studied philosophy at uni, not that he ever completed a full semester. Their parents never understood. Hard working emigrants from the north of England, a bricklayer and a nurse, they were suspicious of his impassioned rants on meaning, consciousness, Heidegger, Nietzsche and the decline of Western civilisation.

'Just get yourself a trade, son, then you can mess around with all this philosophy malarkey in your spare time,' Dad would say, and Pete would roll his eyes at Helen.

In the living room she straightened books and magazines, wiped dust off the coffee table. Like he'd care. If he did notice, he'd only be scathing about her conventional middle-aged sensibilities. 'God, you're just like Mum,' he'd say and it wouldn't be from familial fondness.

It had really been his time. The mid-eighties, their share house days, when uni was free and deeply held political conviction was so much more important than money. Back then, a party without Pete lacked something - a frisson, a certain kind of energy. He challenged people, got them thinking. He would perch on the arm of a crum- bling sofa, a crowd around him sitting cross-legged on the floor, as he argued, disclaimed, lectured, his eyes shining and arms tracing big arcs to make his point.

'Get off your soapbox mate,' one of the guys not enthralled by Pete's barrage of words would call out from across the room, 'Just chill out and have a drink.'

She winced as the familiar guilt crept up on her, remembering anew it was she, the older sister, who had passed him the first beer, his first spliff. But everyone was doing it then, and they were all experi- menting with harder stuff. She and Pete took acid together, had tried ecstasy, but the loss of control had frightened her. Helen had quickly left it all behind for study, for stability. Meanwhile he had flung himself headfirst into a downward spiral of drugs, booze, pills. A vortex from which he seemed unable to escape, decades on.

She stopped abruptly. Maybe he's ready to quit again? Maybe that's why he is coming back to me? He needs me!

Helen sat on the couch. She felt shaky. Could she do it again? Could she support Pete to quit one more time? She couldn't even count how many times she had driven him to rehab, visited him daily and witnessed the grinding pain of withdrawal, seen him emerge fresh and clear eyed, newly determined to stay clean. In all those years, in all those attempts, he'd never even made it to three months.

Helen liked to be needed. Could even say she lived to be needed. In moments of self-aware clarity she realised this desire in her had driven her towards social work. But she was also certain she did not lack genuine empathy. Her ex used to joke (unkindly, she had come to realise, and this dawning understanding had helped fuel their sepa- ration) that her empathy gland was as overactive as her thyroid. Her ex would beg her not to visit the markets because she always came back with unwanted crafts and jars of jam they never ate, thanks to her disproportionate sympathy for the stallholders with no custom- ers.

It was her empathy which had led her to keep trying, long after her parents had tearfully given up. She'd given Pete money, food, beds to sleep in. She had dropped care packages to his latest boarding house, paid for a mobile phone plan for a while, anything to keep him tied to her in some small way. But he continued to slip further and further away from her, until he seemed beyond help and out of her reach. St Jude, the patron saint of lost causes. Dad had called her that for a while until any mention of Pete was too painful for all of them.

She slumped back into the couch. I'm getting too old for this shit. Just the thought of helping Pete through another detox drained her. If she let it, all of her energy could seep out of her, into the plush leather couch, to leave her limp. But she had made no promises yet. It was just one night.

She stood up. Walked across the room to the shelves. It was second nature now to place anything valuable and portable out of sight. She had long ago erased the mental tally of all the money Pete owed her, or later, when things got worse, how much he'd stolen from her. Better to put temptation out of the way. She moved the silver teapot that had belonged to their grandmother. The ivory and mahogany mah-jong set from her own trip to Malaysia. The antique Tibetan prayer bowl. She held the copper bowl in her left palm, and moved the smooth wooden mallet around and around the rim. It sang to her. An eerie, harmonic tone. She had bought it on a trip she and Pete had made to Dharamsala, decades ago, back when all he did was pot. Their visit had coincided with the Dalai Lama's annual teach- ings. They went to the enormous monastery, where the Dalai Lama sat small and distant in front of a sea of monks draped in maroon and saffron. Helen and Pete were grouped with all the other back- packers in a special section where the lectures were translated into halting English. All the impatient Westerners had hoped for easy, instant enlightenment, but instead received quite detailed instruc- tion on how to arrange an altar for daily devotions. So everyone had eventually slipped away to go drink chai in the cafés.

She shook her head. He should be here soon.

She set the table with placemats, knives and forks, even two candles. She squirmed, a wave of physical discomfort coursed through her when she remembered the last time she and Pete had sat at a table together for a meal. Could it really be four years ago? When both their parents were still alive and the dinner table was awash with quiet desperation. All three of them, she, Mum and Dad, convinced that if Pete didn't get help soon, go into rehab one more time, he'd be forever lost to them. They had used every weapon they had at their disposal that night: bribes, incentives, anger, sadness, kindness, all manner of emotion- al blackmail. But it was doomed. What had they been thinking? Of course Pete would feel ambushed. He had exploded. Shoved the table into the bellies of his parents opposite him, flung plates and glasses on the floor, at the walls, where streaks of tomato passata stained the wall for weeks.

'None of you bastards understand,' Pete had screamed in her face on his way out the door. 'Just get off my fucking case.'

She put the glassware at the back of the cupboard. Must dig out those picnic tumblers. She didn't necessarily anticipate a violent outburst but her glasses were new and expensive and she wasn't going to risk it. She'd serve them both sparkling water. It would do her good not to drink her usual couple of glasses of red over dinner.

It had been hard though, not to open a bottle of wine while she cooked. It was her after-work ritual, a way to decompress after a diffi- cult day. Crank the music up loud, make a simple healthy dinner for one and wash it all down with half a bottle of Shiraz. Maybe just one glass, before he gets here, just to chill out a bit. Everything is done now. She would brush her teeth before he arrived.

Wine in hand she opened the oven to check on dinner. She had decided on vegetarian lasagne and salad for its nutritional value. Even if it were only for one night, she was determined to get the maximum amount of vitamins into him. The cheese on top of the lasagne was perfectly melted and browned, and she turned the oven off. The digital clock glowed 6:56. She had told him 7pm but who knew when he might arrive. She still wasn't convinced he would arrive at all. She put the glass down and placed both hands on the gleaming granite benchtop. Her heart fluttered and leapt into her throat.

The buzzer. He was on time. Early even. When had Pete ever, in his entire life, been early for anything? And she hadn't even cleaned her teeth. She quickly rinsed the glass, swilled some water around in her mouth and put the wine at the back of the cupboard. She pressed the button to let him in the front gate. Turned on the front light, breathed deeply then opened the door.

She looked straight into a soft, round glowing face with clear blue eyes made more prominent by the close shaven head. She had to peer closer to confirm this really was her brother. Robes. He wore maroon and saffron robes, with one shoulder exposed. It's a cool night, won't he be cold? It was an irrational thought, she knew that, but she was so confused.

'Pete?' she shook her head. Looked away then back. It really was him.

He had always had beautiful eyes, and now they looked at her with such love that it made her own eyes well up. It was through this haze of tears that she watched Pete take her hands in both of his. He squeezed them hard, looked straight into her eyes and said 'Forgive me.'

We Caught Her In the Act

Kate Cantrell

She said it started at Adam's party and ended in New Farm Park. She came to school the Monday after with half a bottle of vodka and bruises on her arms. She said they were laughing and playing The Killers. It was light when the garbo found her. You asked what happened next. The paramedics came to assess her situation. They checked her pulse and her breathing, then wrapped her in up Al-foil. You grabbed her wrist. We should tell someone, you said. I suggested her sister, Laura. No, she said, Laura was just a kid. And, besides, it was sorted. She was going to the clinic after school. She just needed some cash. Between us we had $11. It wasn't much but we gave her what we had. She counted the gold coins into towers then she knocked them down and stacked them up again. Eventually, the bell rang and Sister Elvera appeared at the chapel window. We stood up quickly and fixed our skirts. She nodded as we passed.

Two weeks later, there was a fire in the science lab. Mr. Newton acci- dentally mixed sugar with potassium nitrate which caused a small explosion. We lined up on the tennis court while the fireys checked the building. She pointed at the oldest. He's not bad, she said, I'd blow him for a smoke. I pretended not to hear. What about Adam? you said. She shrugged. The building was cleared. The fireys returned with their yellow helmets and portable extinguishers. She called out to the one she liked: show us your dick. He turned around and grinned. His black hair was starting to grey and he bulged over his belt. He grabbed his dick and pretended to wank it. When they left he blew the horn.

In winter, a rumour went around that a girl in Grade 10 was pregnant. For some reason, this upset her. Fucking Catholics, she said. She started to skip class. We caught her in the chapel, one day, smoking pot behind the organ. I was angry but we owed her. That's what you said. We sat, cross-legged, on the mosaic floor. Her dress was faded and ripped at the hem and her shoes were threaded with rainbow laces instead of the standard black. Her pot was in a pencil case that she'd labelled Miraculous Cannabis. She wanted us to try it. She rolled the joint between her lips and lit the end. You took the joint reluctantly and examined it. It's like smoking a cigarette, she said, but you hold it in your lungs as long as you can. You puffed a few times and started to cough.

A haze of smoke appeared between us. You're wasting it, she said. You apologised and she snatched it from your hand. I stood near the holy water and kept watch for Sister. She relit the joint. You know Sister's a lesbian, she said. She took a long draw. I saw her with Sister Cecil in the city last weekend. You're lying, I said. She laughed and blew smoke rings at the Virgin Mary.

Months passed. Spring returned from wherever it disappeared to and the jacarandas bloomed. The jets flew over at Riverfire. We passed our final exam. Then, one morning at the vending machine, she told us what happened. There were four of them. Five, if you included the first one, but she struggled so much in the beginning he couldn't get it up. The rest waited in line for their turn. They had team spirit, she said. She sipped her Coke. I wanted to know how long she fought. You wanted her to forgive us. If we could go back, we'd call Adam and tell him to fuck off. We'd have been there, you said. We'd have taken you with us. She shook her head. It's better it was me, she said. She lit another cigarette and blew the smoke over her shoulder. We asked if she would quit. She said she wasn't sure. She didn't believe in the afterlife but she thought there was another world after Death. A world where you don't need your body, she said.

The next day, she withdrew her statement at the station. I can't go to court, she said. She asked us to paint our fingernails black, you know, in solidarity. I thought it was a strange request but we did it anyway. What else could we do? You were afraid she'd leave us forever and I was too busy opening the chapel windows to let in some air.

By the time Christmas came around, she'd started talking about Evanescence. The band's lead singer was a Goth who described herself as a dirty slut. She copied the words onto her graduation certificate when her parents weren't looking. It's not an insult, she said. I asked her what she meant. She said, if you want to offend a guy then you call his mum a slut. There's no male equivalent for a guy who's a whore. It's the same in every language. She paused for a moment to see if I was getting it. It's a double standard, I said. She shook her head. It's more than that. She seemed to think the differ- ence between good and bad was only a matter of perspective.

In the New Year you went to Fiji with your cousin and I developed asthma. The papers said there was too much pollen in the air. A botanist came on the news and said this is what happens when there are too many male plants. Males, he said, don't produce seed pods or messy fruits, but, with so many around, the pollen they release just hangs in the air waiting for us to inhale it. We should ban male plants, he said. His colleague agreed: it's better to grow plants with both male and female parts. I called, tired and wheezy, to tell you we should blame the men. You laughed and said you'd met a guy called Jesh. He was a Hindu but he didn't force it on anyone. You were taking him to your cousin's wedding. You were choosing his kurta. My breath left without warning. I became aware of my heart.

In February, we agreed to meet at Sizzlers for lunch but you never showed. We called you twice but your phone was off. We waited in the restaurant until everyone went home and the manager asked us to leave. On the way out she stole a beer. For my troubles, she said.

That night, I had an asthma attack. I was lying on my bed, thinking about nothing in particular, when my chest clenched up. Mum drove me to the plaza. Doctor McCauley called us into his office and said we needed to get rid of the cat. Mum stared at me. Then she turned to Doctor McCauley and said, we've had Basil longer than she's had asthma. He looked at her blankly. I could hear the clock ticking on the wall above my head. I imagined there was a giant ear pressed to his surgery door. Finally, Mum said, what about an air filter? Would that work? My friend, Jill, got one for her Stedman. Yes, I spose we'll try that. Doctor McCauley spun around in his chair until he was facing his computer. She needs to know her triggers, he said. He folded a sheet of paper in half and scribbled 'Internal' on the front and 'External' on the back. He handed me a pen. Triggers are things that irritate your airways and make you feel worse. I clicked the pen once and wrote: smoking, dust, and animals with fur. Mum objected. But Basil has hair, she said. Doctor McCauley cleared his throat. Fur is a type of hair, he said. Mum patted my knee. She turned to the doctor and said, she can be dramatic, you see. He mumbled some- thing I didn't hear. Then he wrote me a prescription for a special puffer which he called a blue reliever. This is your first line of defence, he said. He pressed the canister to release a clear spray of medicine. I kept the puffer in my bra. When I felt an attack coming on I told myself it would pass. With practice, I learned to breathe through my nose instead of my mouth.

In April, you returned to Fiji and this time you came home with a henna tattoo and two mangled plants. Kava, you said, but I thought you said, carve her. We snuck into the storeroom before school. I sat on the bench and ate grapes while you searched for a knife. Why am I here? she said. She was smoking again. You removed the plants from your backpack and arranged them under a fluorescent light. You cut the roots from the stem. Together, we ground the roots into a thick brown pulp. Then you strained the muddy water through a sieve and offered her a drink. It's for the flashbacks, you said. She raised the bowl to her lips and sipped. It will help, I said. She spat out a mouthful and said, fuck you guys. Then she left. I emptied the bowl into the sink.

That afternoon, she was caught in the chapel with Adam and expelled. We cleared her locker. You kept her Volleys and her green hoodie. I threw her smokes in the bin.

In November, we graduated and went to Schoolies. The girl in Grade 10 had a baby. You went to uni to study art and I signed up for an asthma trial in Sydney. You called sometimes to say you missed her and where was she anyway? You couldn't sleep at night. You kept dreaming you were sitting in a chair, paralysed, as a herd of bulls came stampeding towards you. You would blink your eyes for help, and sometimes turn your head to the sound, but in the end, you were always crushed.

Five years later, she called to say it never happened. There was no party, no paramedics. She saw the Al-foil thing on SVU. She was trying to get clean. She'd been thinking for a while she should tell us the truth. She was high right now but she wasn't drunk. She'd remember this in the morning. I sat down on the bathroom floor and sucked on my inhaler. Where are you? I said. There was a pause followed by a snort. Where are you? I said again. Before she hung up she said she was sorry. It was a long time ago and we'd all changed a lot.

That night, I cancelled my plans for dinner and caught a cab to your house. You were sitting on the verandah watching a magpie swoop. She's sick, I said. She's a fucking sicko. You opened a bottle of red. The cork crumbled. You reached for my hand. We were kids, you said. And, anyway, her dad was a creep. You filled our glasses to the brim. So, we should forgive her, I said. Is that what you're saying? My hands were shaking. I stood up from the table and walked over to the railing. Your children—two boys and a girl—were playing in the garden. I figured

Jesh was in his studio somewhere, tuning a guitar. You joined me on the balcony and put your arms around my waist. We watched as the magpie flew away. Why can't you let go, you said. I felt your breath on my neck. You're drunk again, I said. You threw our empty glasses in the sink and called out to your kids. They picked up their toys from the yard and climbed the stairs, one by one. The youngest was carrying a plastic gun. She's a baddie, he said, pointing at his sister. We caught her in the act. Before I left, you gave me her address.

Saviour

Joshua Wildie

There are two rules a girl like me should live by. Always know your dealer and only take what you can handle. Problem is, the people who've heard these rules a zillion times are exactly the ones who forget about them. Slips their minds so gradually, they don't even notice.

Thought I knew my dealer. Wasn't buddies with the bloke. Didn't even know his real name. Was brought to his street corner by the fella I fancied and I'd been coming back since. What can I say? The product was good and his price was fair. His chit-chat was the sort you get from cashiers. Mundane shit like the weather or how he liked my hair today. Expecting nothing more than a 'not too bad' or 'can't complain' to his 'how are yous?' He never offered up any specifics about himself. Nothing about a missus or friends. Not even if he preferred coffee or tea. I wasn't any better if we're being straight. He'd lean in to hear me mumble my order to my shoelaces and then compliment me on my manners when I said please. He might've been taking the piss but I couldn't help being polite. If habits weren't hard to break, they wouldn't be habits.

Our relationship was all business and I reckon that was fine by both of us. But the personal always barges in on business eventually. I saw him staring at my belly, watching it grow week by week. How much did he know? How well did my dealer know me? More to the point, how well did he know my fella?

The fella who stole my heart told me I was too beautiful to suffer. That he wouldn't want to live in a world where an angel like me could feel pain. We laid naked on a stained mattress in a graffiti-coated room. The smashed windows covered over with cardboard. A field of rubbish across the floor. A glass pipe beside him, blackened from overuse. We were in such a world where girls like yours truly suffer but I kept it to myself. In the moonlit room, I could see his teeth were semi-translucent. His skin worn beyond his twenty-something years. His doe-eyes were sinking into an abyss they'd never come back from. The fact his beauty was visibly fleeting made him all the more gorgeous. I saw decay in him but he saw me as his saviour.

The last I saw him before he went AWOL, it was dawn. I awoke and found him still unconscious. When I touched his bristled neck I felt a dull thud through my fingertips. I found my clothes, got dressed and left. Didn't leave a number or nothing. We always seemed to bump into each other and I just assumed that routine would continue. My head was in the toilet for the third day in a row when I twigged I'd no way of contacting him. Just didn't seem cool not to tell him. Problem was, he had no home and mobile phones freaked him out. Some- thing about the cops listening in or the like. Finding my fella was like remembering a dream. The harder you try, the hazier every detail gets. But there was someone who might've been able to help me find him. A mutual acquaintance.

For weeks, months even, I kept finding my dealer on his corner. Arriving with good intentions, leaving with easy answers. I always said I could stop when it became too much but when it became too much I only knew one solution. His 'how are yous' felt more urgent. He started to squeeze my shoulder. But then things fell into place. I'd ask what he was holding. The pitch flowed from his lips with a tired precision. He'd always take my money and hook me up. Without meeting his eyes, I'd search his face, his stance, the words he spoke for any evidence he knew where my fella was. The idea of asking him scared the shit out of me.

Each time I walked away I'd promise it'd be the last time. I'd go home, make things right with my parents. Get help. For real this time. But I'd keep finding myself on the corner. I'd keep waking up in restrooms, abandoned houses and alleyways. Not getting high anymore. More like plateauing.

When we were together, my fella would have moments of whimsy. He'd talk about us and our future. He wanted to buy a car. Nothing fancy. Just something to get us from A to any letter in the alphabet we liked. We'd be free of the system. No rent. No boss breathing down our neck. Just the two of us. We'd do odd jobs to survive. Fruit picking and the like. We could fall asleep snuggling in the backseat every night. It was going to happen. He promised to take me away from all this.

He was telling me his plans while sitting cross-legged in just his undies, waving a flame under a spoon. With a syringe in his mouth, he mumbled that he knew a guy who knew a guy who had an old Commo- dore he was looking to pawn off. Real cheap. Like only five hundred bucks and my fella reckoned he could talk him down from that.

'Do you have that kind of money?'

He began pulling back the plunger and the needle drank the fluid from the spoon. He answered, 'Oh Angel, I often got that kinda money, but you know that kinda money has a ways of slipping through a person's fingers, don't it?'

Drops came from the end of the needle as he flicked it and examined the barrel for air.

'I've never done it like this before,' I said. 'Maybe we should stick to what we know.'

'She'll be right, Angel. Like, you might feel a bit shitty at some point. Just stay calm and it'll pass. Once you get over that hurdle, it'll be all peaches and gravy. You'll be free in a way you've never been before.'

'Like when you buy this car, huh?'

'Bingo. We're going to be okay, okay? Trust me.'

He handed me the end of his belt to hold in my teeth. The leather tight around my arm. The buckle dug into my skin while my fella found a vein.

Before he pressed down, he kissed my forehead. His smile exposed the sadness it was trying to hide. He told me I had the most beautiful eyes, like the deer in that Disney movie. My body went limp and my tongue liquefied before I could tell him the name of the film.

Whenever my eyes close, I see him. I see him lying in alleyways. Sometimes with broken bones, bleeding out into the gutter. His pockets turned inside out. His shoes taken only to make the beating worth something. Most of the time I see him in desolate buildings, parks, public toilets, emergency rooms or in the house of someone he's just given his last dollar to. His shirt covered in vomit. His skin grey. Arms festered with sores. Eyes extinguished.

Beautiful people don't leave beautiful corpses. Death doesn't discriminate.

My brush with optimism is the same scenario but his legs hang out the backseat of a crappy Holden Commodore. The fourth-rate paint job not coming close to hiding the rust. The police at the scene may shake their heads and the public may hold it up as evidence of kids these days but not me. Him trying and failing was better than empty promises lost in the ether. A sign he died there and not long ago.

My fella's vehicular coffin faded and I woke up on a park bench. A little boy greeted me and asked my name and I told him before asking his. Before he answered, his mum ran up and grabbed him. The disgust she wore melted when I looked up and met her eyes. She asked how old I was. I added a few years and told her I was nineteen. Rummaging in her purse, she found a twenty and held it out to me.

'Don't waste it all, love,' she said.

I told her I'd buy food. She shook her head.

'Forget about the money. If you could see what I see, you'd stop what you're doing.'

I nodded. The note fluttered in my shaking fingers. 'Thank you,' I said.

She and her son left hand in hand. I watched them board a bus and leave. Time's a concept I'd given up a while ago but I know I was on that bench for a while. There was a playground crawling with children. Some hung from the monkey bars. Others climbed up the slide. A few swung back and forth on the swings. The present is so lovely when the future doesn't interfere.

With the afternoon sun in my eyes, I felt a kick inside me. I put my hand under my shirt in time for the next one. My heart raced. I had the most beautiful anxiety attack. Feeling high in a way I hadn't for so long. Like I might OD.

My body spasmed. The smile that broke through my face felt like a discovery. My cheeks were warm when I wiped away the tears. I held my belly with both hands. Every kick shook my world.

The train home didn't depart for a few more minutes. My blood crawled in my veins. I stopped grinding my teeth, only to bite the inside of my cheeks until they bled. A layer of cold sweat coated my skin. My eyeballs shivered. Withdrawal was an aggressive fever dream I couldn't wake up from. And my fella was still missing. And the kicks kept on coming. More than I could handle.

Out the window, a heart-shaped helium balloon caught my eye. The string led to a little girl who was laughing at her father's antics. She hugged his legs, letting go of her balloon. When her father turned to catch it, I met the eyes of my dealer for the first time. He squinted at me. He pressed a finger to his lips then ran it across his throat. He then gave me a sad smile and a shrug. Next second, he handed the balloon to his daughter and was back to being her goofy Dad. As the train left the city behind, I finally got it. He wasn't making a threat. It was a plea. Please, don't find out what happens if you mention my loved ones to the wrong people. Not a choice but a necessity. For his family, he'd end mine before it began.

Maybe there was still a chance the dealer would help me track down my fella. But as I slipped in and out of sleep, I realised I wasn't too fussed on finding him. Or seeing the dealer again. Not yet. I couldn't trust myself around either man. The wheels clicked beneath the gently swaying carriage. Looking out the window, I thought about my fella leaning against his shitbox of a car outside some servo out in the middle of nowhere. Drinking a cold coke while looking out the desert landscape. The blank canvas he'd always wanted waiting for him to scrawl across. When we meet in the next life I'll have to ask him whether I'm the fingerprint on his brain that he is on mine.

I slouched in my chair, rubbed my once-flat stomach, and prayed for a miracle. Maybe this was something I could handle. Whatever it took. Throwing whoever I had to under the train. Believing in the slivers of hope I could grasp. Maybe it wasn't too late to save myself. To save us.

End of Lease

Elspeth Ives

Further to the End of Lease instructions forwarded 24 December 2016, attached is an updated list of items needing attention. These were recorded during your Landlord's recent property inspection.

A friendly reminder that return of bond to the Tenant is condi- tional upon the property being left in the same state it was in at the commencement of lease, 23 December 2010.

1. Garage must be emptied.

Dispersed among the unused rooms at my old place, my belongings didn't seem so numerous. On moving day, in boxes, they pile up like cardboard monuments colonising this empty house and I can't help noticing the imbalance between what we're both contributing to the new partnership. You've borrowed a trailer to bring your stuff here. Removalists huff in the December heat with my possessions, emerging from their truck again and again and maybe I see a shake of your head and your frown lines deepen. I laugh. You said you hated the carpet, now you'll never see it again.

On one box, I've scrawled glassware and nervously filled it with tissue paper, clouded crystal and shallow, saucer-like champagne glasses. I used to watch my grandparents hold them by the stems for celebratory toasts, the gold rims chiming prettily with party guests' jewellery. Once my grandfather had noticed me by his side as he filled a tray-load of these with shimmery liquid and he had pointed to the centre of one of the glasses. Fizzing up from the hollow stem had been a tiny fast-moving marvel, a fountain of silver-gold bubbles. I rescue the glassware box from the top of a stack, unwrap a tissue nest and hold up a glass to you. This stuff is useful.

I position two glasses on the chipped Laminex in the tired kitchen whose faux-cork vinyl floor has smooth patches where feet have stood for decades to wash dishes. The glasses, vessels of gaiety and wonder, promise reward at the end of moving day.

I open boxes gingerly, as if the more gradually everything is revealed, the less you'll realise how much stuff I have. It's hard to be furtive, though, when newspaper accumulates incriminating- ly behind me and oddments from the eras of the entire previous century fill the spaces between the boxes, like ligaments branching out from my hands as they work.

A Noah's Ark of animal figurines prospers on the carpet, bundled silverware forms buttresses against the boxes and several entire dinner sets are yet to be unearthed. Somewhere there are polished wooden cases with velvet depressions clasping silver cutlery. At some point I'll excavate crates of burred papers, files bulging with drawings and writings, letters, cards and postcards between people long gone or forgotten. I stand a shiny ceramic pitcher on the floor and around its capacious middle is a reflected version of me: familiar and peculiar, it has all my features, but the expressionistic distortion is unnerving.

Do you ever feel you're forming the wrong kinds of attachments? You ask with affection but with a disquieting precision. Then you mention the empty garage and I wonder who will give in first.

2. Oven is to be thoroughly cleaned.

New Year's Eve comes a few days after the move. New year, new life. You'd like to cook a meal, just us. You rub my back and give me a look of unreserved love. I feel un undertow, and self-reproach.

Carrying a cooler bag with ice bricks, you take off for an early train, headed to the city market. I wave you off, promising to tackle more boxes. Then I wander up to explore the local shops where I buy three bath mats – one in every available colour – which is a dreary house-warming purchase, so I also pick up a potted jade plant from the supermarket.

You return after lunch, cheeks warm with the heat and the exertion of carrying a cooler bag stretched with vegetables, plump olives and cheeses. You've bought a champagne bottle, portly like a bowling pin, gold tracery on the label. Then with great showmanship, grimacing and straining of muscles, you remove from the bag a giant raw bird. Goose. I think my eyebrows rocket skywards because I've never encountered a goose for cooking before, only the hissing kind strutting around in the dirt with a full complement of feathers.

Your excitement is infectious and I don't want to seem hostile after your odyssey but the goose, supine on the Laminex, vast, yellowish and pimply fails to charge my appetite. The skin and grim recline make me think of a stout naked woman, meaty legs splayed on either side of an ominous cavity, possibly in the act of giving birth. It'll be amazing. I ask if this is something you do, cook geese. Never. We're laughing.

Several hours of mid-summer cooking turn the kitchen into an oily-smelling steam bath. Hot from the oven, the bird's appeal hasn't improved. It overhangs the roasting pan, which is clearly inadequate for a creature of this stature. Its legs – stiffened through cooking – point to opposite corners of the kitchen. A film of sweat on your face, you pull away a goose leg and bend down to peer at the flesh to see whether it's cooked. You shrug and declare it done and I allow the tingling of champagne to dull my distaste.

Our meal hardly dents the bulk of the goose, which goes back into the oven out of range of the circling flies. We carry on with our evening and hear fireworks somewhere distant at midnight. Forgot- ten, the carcass remains in the oven in the heat of several early-Jan- uary days, until it is discovered as the source of a sour fug we can taste on the backs of our tongues. Enshrouded in a fetid pall the largely intact bird, skin deflated, has settled in a bath of satiny-grey congealed fat, a gash in its breast where it was carved. Opening the oven door wide, I can see goose fat has spattered every surface and overflow has pooled on the oven floor. I let the door swing shut on the thick air.

3. Un-rotted compost to be removed from premises.

By the next summer I have taken over the garden and seams of pot plants encroach on the concrete path. The succulents continue their mathematical expansion whether I care for them or not but most of the plastic pots hold husks like spindly grave markers, once-lush horticultural exemplars now withered by neglect and shaggy with weeds.

Now and again I haul pungent manures and sea liquids home from the hardware. Touting nourishment for my garden projects they aid in the cultivation of several artichokes that flower impressively over otherwise fallow beds. Buoyed, I start collecting kitchen scraps in a corroding aluminium basin, tipping them behind the lichened liquidambar. I start referring to the decomposing rodent-attracting mass as the compost bay.

By the third year you are edgy. One morning, grey hairs newly at your temples and wearing a collared work-shirt, you block my way at the back door and pin me with an imploring look. We moved out with a plan. Your tone is exquisitely even, the way it is when you need to stop something from boiling over. I am blank. Are you even worried? I duck around you and fling something conciliatory. It'll happen. Your sigh is audible from the steps. Bullshit. Out under the liquidambar I jab the pitchfork's curved tines into the compost, a ripe batter speckled with variously mouldering bits of peel and panicked worms, overwhelmed by too much of a good thing, suddenly displaced. I push the living sludge around, though it hurts my arms and is bracing to inhale.

4. Any holes in walls to be filled in and re-painted. (Paint to be supplied by Landlord.)

I'm suffused with an unshakeable sense of desire when I spy some- thing good at the shops. The moment I decide to buy is bliss. To fit through the front door I always walk in sideways, both hands loaded with shopping bags, one in front, the other behind. I dump everything on the bed, fingers stinging as they uncurl from the plastic handles. I have another surge of well-being when my new things tumble onto my bed. But then, looking at everything - shirts, shoes, secateurs, pens, plates and god knows what - the onset of dread at the thought of you seeing it all. I'm running out of scope for the constant imperative to arrange things throughout the house to disguise the steady stream of incoming goods.

By the time we've lived together four years I've stuffed the house, garden and garage so I take measurements along one lounge room wall. A delivery day is set for when you're at work and two men spend hours in the lounge room, furniture pushed to the side, putting together a wall-sized unit with moveable shelves and silent-close doors. They spray the whole thing with a skin of glossy white paint. When they position metal brackets along the top of the unit and pick up the drill I remind them we rent. They say they have to affix these things. Kids just see these as climbing frames – you don't want your kids getting crushed by one of these. I tell them No, that I don't.

When you walk in you stop dead, put your knapsack on the couch, then keep walking past me to the bathroom. More of these units could fit in the hall. I take your silence as tacit support for the installation of storage solutions, as the brochure put it. They're a neat way of delineat- ing mine and yours. No need for you to know that when I buy a top, I buy it in every colour – everything's so cheap these days it makes sense if you find something you like and that fits. Never mind the children who've made this stuff, you said once, early on, before I was organised.

5. Flyscreens to be reinstated.

I'm rearranging some pots outside when I see you up a stepladder reaching for the little tabs that hold one of the flyscreens in place. You're not keen on home maintenance so I'm curious. Your move- ments are jerky as you dislodge the flyscreen, come down the ladder and lean the screen against a stack you've already taken out. Then you take a screen in each hand and disappear under the house.

When I approach I see you're flushed and sweating and puffing. You glance at me and continue moving flyscreens under the house. When you're finished, you're wiping your hands on your pant-legs and shaking your head. I'm smothered in that house. Anything to get the air moving. Your eyes are wet. I say you're crazy.

I'm crazy?

6. Broken glass panel in front door to be fixed at Tenant's expense.

Opening the bedroom door I see you standing on a chair and pulling things from a storage unit, sending them down in a cascade of emptying bags. The hallway is a colourful pool of plastic whose retail logos plot my movements over several years. I can't read the expres- sion on your face but you know I'm there. This is not okay.

I feel an acid charge in my body; my heartbeat accelerates through my chest and up into my head firing a heat in my face that spreads down to the ground.

It was always your thing - a baby - not mine. You turn away and when I see the nape of your neck I register a pang. Of love, of loss? I can't tell. You release a bag from your hand, step off the chair and wade along the hallway to walk out the front door, which shatters against the house.

As previously advised in the End of Lease instructions, two property keys must be returned to our office by 5pm on the final day of occupation.

Felidae

He be the only one of the litter who lives. I wraps the tiny stillborn bodies in the bloody cloth she birthed them on an carries them out. She rolls way from the muck an pain of it an I takes up the last one in my paws, his skin slick with her insides, so little the curve of his back cups in the fold of my palm. I blows gently on his nostrils, clearing the blood way for the air. I sees how much of my Aidan is in him already: the slanty face, the tawny eyes. I puts my tongue gainst the strip of fur growin down his back an drags it long the length of his body, tastin her blood. She turns to watch me, pushin herself up in them damp sheets, her body tremblin. I holds the cub out to her, his tiny paws with them human fingers curled.

'You had better be givin him a feedin. Don't want no mewlin from the wee thing.'

He wiggles in my hands, the blood dryin sticky on his pinky skin. She takes him an holds him gainst her chest, his teeth needle at her nipples, sharp an fierce. She looks fraid, like all new ness do, an I puts my paw gainst her face, wipin way the sweat an tears, kissin her tangled hair.

'You call him Leo, like the big lion in the stars.'

It were after curfew; the streets be burnin, bright an still. The heat frightnin big, a white wall that falls on you, pressin down on you, the air dry as an old bone. She dragged her moon body through them streets, probably never been outside with the sun up before, too hot to breathe. In the Cradle, the streets a narrow mess of tin walls, slum place where only Feli lives, she came to find us. Her own pride didn't want nothin to do with her after Aidan. JemBoy didn't want to takes her in at first, she from under the ground where the unmixed lives, but I growl him down.

'She a mother of cub. We gone help her. You wanna be like them, decidin who worthy of help?'

After the baby comes, we keeps her shut away. The water gone, after that last war there ain't be nothing left – them desal plants burned and bombed. Canberra shut itself in behind them walls an now them po-man don't come up the Cradle too much no more, too hot an Feli been no bothers for some while, but never can be too careful. I seen them once rip a cub from a ness an cracks his skull open on the hard dusty ground, leavin ness wailin while them stomp away in them heat tectin suits. Somethins be worse than death for us though.

Redmond Park. In my dreams I presses my body gainst the wire, my voice keenin his name in the burnin air. There be blood on the dust. Them pulls out his claws with pliers, his teeth. I can smells rot; them line them up gainst the walls an don't bury them after. The nesses holds the cubs up gainst the fences for mercy, beggin, cryin. But them hates the halfies most of all.

'You gotta run, girl. You aint know what them do to him, you aint seen. Your Aidan, he done. An you done too now; you got cub. You wanna keep that boy? You run. Them take him out to that island with the others an you ain't never see him gain.'

I thinks of Aidan's hands, them cut an broke paws he'd ruined to try an be more like them, to try an hide what he is. His body a mess of pearly scars, crooks in the Cradle tell you them make you look human by cuttin you. Aint no way we ever gone look like them. I looks down at the baby sleepin in her arms, an knows that no matter what them will only ever see the lion in him.

'We try get you out. Take you out in the Pilbara.' 'The desert.'

She knows what it mean. All that red earth an not a drop of water left. 'Them can't follow you out there.'

Leo wriggles in her arms. She touch his feline face with her fingertips an he yawns, wide, his tiny sharp teeth bright in the dark.

'Them put a bag over your head an shoot you dead for what you done.'

She looks long in my eyes, an I sees she knows she dead either way. But she nods an kisses the baby, breathin him in. At least this way him have a chance.

We have to go at night, it's too damn hot in the day for her, that sun blisterin in the thin air, under that hole in the sky. Feli don't feel nuthin, we made to be outside. Them put us up here to do what them couldn't, but it make no difference now. She swallows the water tabs desperately; Leo's greedy sucklin tears the moisture from her. His face different to mine an Jemboy, got the looks of her well as Aidan. I sees her wonderin.

'It don't always come out the same. We Felidae, we all be different. When them were muckin about with all those genes, them didn't know what them were playin at. Didn't think we'd be able to breed none.' Her skin is so dry it's peelin, salty sheets raspin off. The tabs keep her from dryin out, but only barely. I reckon them hates us partly cause we free from the need of water; that's why them made us an now them hates us for it.

'Do you have any children Gammy?'

I thinks about Aidan, mostly mine but not from inside.

'No baby of mine live. I not born, I made. Cook in tube, little cat fish in glass. Not thirsty no, but damn lot a good it do me. I never been loved by a human man, an nothin Feli make mongst ourselves ever come out breathin.'

JemBoy worryin she gone cause trouble for all us, he chewin on it— he have good reason be fraid. His ness in the Park now, good as dead. He don't want no one come lookin for her.

'Where your people girl?'

Her voice flat like the land outside, dry an dead. I knows the story. 'They lived in the Heather Compound. After Aidan, they didn't

want to see me anymore. They didn't believe in integration.' JemBoy huffs a harsh sound.

'And then them baby girl got Pride.'

I thinks bout how it were before the fences went up. I remembers the rallies, some them wanted us allowed. Them chanted in the streets, not human, still people, but the candles go out when the gas fall on them. Everythin turns hazy in the stingin fog, people screamin, eyes burnin. The po-man press gainst the crowds with them shields, herding them back. The banners go down, those peace wantin words trodden gainst the dirt. The screamin gets louder when the bones begin to break, them evil black sticks smashin gainst the ones who push back. I thinks bout her ma, the dried husk of her body after the compound breached an them rebels took the water. Her pappa, on his knees, cold metal in his mouth. Justice maybe, for all he done.

'Did you knows them were gonna takes him?'

She turns to me, lookin at me with them blue eyes he couldn't keeps way from. I feels my voice hard, fur bristlin down my back. The reason Aidan in the Park be that baby sleepin in her arms.

'I'm sorry Gammy. I loved him. I wanted to believe they would understand that, that they could see him the way I do.'

I'm growlin, for a minute I lose all the words them never wanted me to have. But I thinks bout how he'd come home sometimes after, all lit like, how she made him see that he weren't an animal to all of them.

'Him loved you too.'

JemBoy says we gotta leave, we been careful but we all knows them ain't gonna let it go – Aidan in the Park but the po-man don't want no halfies goin free. Them comin for that cub, sure as sure. We almost out of the sight of the Cradle, it disappearing into the night behind us and there's just open sand front of us, when I hears it.

There's a bright moon an the dunes are licked blue in the moon- light. JemBoy roars at me, he off over the sand but I runs back toward her, so fraid I can feel my heart tearin in me.

'Take Leo!'

She holds the cub out to me, her limbs thin like sticks. I puts my claws in her flesh.

'You comin with us girl!'

She rips her arm from me an pushes the cub gainst my body. 'Take him.'

We looks at each other, the whap whap of the copter beatin the sand round us into the air, can't breathe none. I takes her in my arms, an kisses her with my whiskery mouth.

'I ain't never let them find him. Him gone be free.'

She's cryin, the last water she got fallin gainst my fur. Taking the cub by his scruff in my mouth, I puts all four paws gainst the hot earth an I runs. I looks back once and sees her on her knees with them lights shinin on her, watchin as I carries her son away over the sand, into the desert dark.

When them puts the black bag over her head, I is long gone.

Twin Suns

James McKenzie Watson

We grew up in a weatherboard house twelve kilometres from town. Lone structure in a bare paddock, distant border of scrub in each direction. It shimmered on the horizon like a marble mirage when the dusk caught it properly. Gold against the bruised blues and purples of the earth's shadow. A ship of gleaming, ethereal light navi- gating a beige and listless sea.

It was built almost a century ago before suffering a series of haphazard transformations outwards and upwards. Rooms and floors tacked on here and there. Verandas insulated by ceilings and walls to form draughty hallways. Cold in the central spaces of the ground floor, even in summer.

The five of us could've each had our own room—enough space for a dozen families in that house—but, for whatever reason, we chose not to. Sally and dad shared the centre bedroom by the kitchen until Sally was fourteen when she moved to one of the newer, second floor rooms. John, Boyd and I were in the master bedroom right up to the day John died. Three single beds lined beneath a vast window that looked out over the eastern paddock and the grey-green blur of scrub beyond. Two horizons, the tide of bush at the plain's end and the void of the heavens above that. During summer's apex, the sky there would be a blue so pale it was no longer a colour. The atmos- phere's false hue exposed as though we had an unfiltered view into the cosmos. Space isn't black and cold and formless. It's the harshest white you've ever known.

We never moved John's bed, the middle one, out of the room after he died. It stayed there, gathering dust, a physical wedge between Boyd and I that pried like a jack iron until we were so distant from one another we may as well have been living on different planets.

I didn't know I was going to burn the house down until the day I did it. I don't even think it was my idea. Someone else put it in my head. Plucked it out of the barren soil and planted it in my brain. Nourished it with kinetic energy, the throb of my heartbeat harnessed and utilised. I wasn't sure where I'd light the fire, just knew it had to be somewhere it'd spread quickly. Couldn't be Sally's sanctuary—no real structural connection to the rest of the building. Her room could be reduced to a pile of ash, lapping against the next wall with each breath of wind, and you wouldn't know about it from the other side of the house. Dad's wouldn't work either—too much cement, not enough to catch. In the end, as much as I disliked the idea, it was clear that the master bedroom was the only option. Central enough that a fire would weaken the beams and cripple the rest of the beast. I resigned myself to this actuality despite my misgivings. I didn't like the idea of setting light to where John died. Felt like I was killing him all over again.

Boyd and dad were out in the paddocks when I did it. Hunting in the shadows of dawn while the world was ataxic with the cold. I thought Sally was with them but I guess she was still in bed. I misjudged how much petrol I'd need and lost my eyebrows when I struck the match.

Out into that sea of wild grass as the house erupted, great ribbons of flame embracing the roof and reaching serpentine coils through exploding windows. Pillar of black smoke rising, a distress call to other ships on this vast ocean. I whooped and cheered and dived through the fields as the sun rose behind the house, a second orb at the horizon, a twin to my blaze.

I knew the moment dad and Boyd burst from the scrub, their voices shredding as they screamed for Sally, their palms raised against the heat, that I'd messed up. Obvious that I probably wouldn't get away with it that time. But Christ, it's not like there was anything else to do out there.

A Belt for Buddha

Paul Mitchell

I punched an abandoned factory's brick walls every night with my bare hands for practice.

All right, my hands weren't completely bare; I stuck cut out bits from a hessian bag on them.

The walls were the colour of month-old dog shit and I drove down to the factory on my way home from work. It was near the Maribyrnong, on the other side from the Buddhist Temple and the giant statue of the gold Buddha or whatever. It was the old Franken First National Factory where they used to make money. Literally. The yard smelt like wet horse hair mixed with petrol, but I liked its walls better than the empty Matteck Mill's walls next-door. Franken's had knotty lumps in them. Something to aim at. I danced and sparred and watched the statue, shining quiet and peaceful even on dull days.

While I punched the living shit out of the Franken walls. Maybe I didn't go at it that hard.

But it was hard enough to rip the skin off my knuckles. If I wasn't drawing blood I wasn't doing it properly. I got callouses after a few months and when I put the MMA gloves on and hit a bloke in full sparring he wouldn't get up in a hurry. And when he did, he'd leave the ring.

I only boxed before MMA. I would have stuck with it, but MMA had bigger crowds. I loved a bit of cheering, especially from the women. There were more of them at MMA, front row seats. It was the new trendy sport then so there was a free glass of champers on entry at some places.

I could box, kick and wrestle. In the end, I wrestled best. Really learnt how to do it nicely. I loved the wrestling tactics, all the ways you had to shift your legs and arms and torso to keep your opponent down.

But I wasn't hard enough when I started. My first bout was a disaster. The bloke was skinnier than me, but he was all technique. It was an amateur bout, but he was all pro; ten years older than me, at least, and he had slick black hair and a tatt on his left tit. Don't know what it was. Maybe some kind of bird? The way I fought that night he'd have had time to get one tattooed on his other tit while I was trying to kick him. I never even got him to the canvas to wrestle. He fucked me up, broke my nose. Nasty shit.

Second bout I won by a lucky knock out. Vietnamese bloke slipped and I caught him with a straight right. Lights out.

I didn't lose another bout before I retired. And I used my nickname, 'The Doc', which I got on account of the legal brothel I was running then. Doctor Feelgood, hey? They asked me to go do the circuit in the US of A and be the Aussie Maltese wog warrior.

No way. Those bastards would have eaten me alive. Or dead.

Whichever came first after they'd turned my head into pizza.

I had to belt a kid at work. I know I shouldn't have done it, I'd been told a hundred thousand times:

You're one of our best youth workers, Doc, so don't go turning it all arse up by belting one of the kids

Then, after I'd done it:

We know it was self-defence, but you could have just ducked.

You try ducking! You try not belting a kid in the guts when he's coming at you with the sole of a runner in your face going for the flying Bruce Lee kick.

Jesus Christ, I'm only human.

Not sure the kids are though. It's a school for drop outs, the ones other schools won't take. Doesn't mean I have to take crap from them though. Not a Bruce Lee amount anyway.

Bosses sacked me. For three months. Bit of leave so I could sort myself out. So I took off to a Buddhist monastery in Bendigo.

Why the fuck not? Get some country air. Bosses wanted me to calm down so I said, Right, I'll show you how much the job means to me. I'll piss off to a monastery and get some good old peace and love.

Yeah, right.

It was hard work. Crazy shit goes down at monasteries.

First off, they won't step on any ants. Whenever I stood on one, they looked at me like I was a rapist. Talked about sentient beings and shit. Jesus, what do you do with people like that? I mean, they're ants! There's squin-billions of them all over the planet, stuffing up picnics and wrecking the Jesus out of honey jars. If I knock off a couple, what's the issue?

The wheel of life, a monk told me. A spread of hair was just starting to grow back on his tanned, bald head. He was Asian. Proper monk.

'Wheel of freakin life?'

'Yes, Doc. It's a cycle. And you may return as an ant.' 'A fucking ant? Why?'

He laughed and sat down on a big rock. Smoothed his brown robe.

'Doc,' he said, 'we must get to the heart of the matter.' 'And what's that?'

'Why you are so angry?'

'I'm not! It's just that when kids throw flying kicks at me I'm going to make sure my face doesn't get pizzerised.'

The monk laughed again.

'Pizza? We don't eat it. I used to like it.' 'How long have you been here?'

We were at the arse-end of the compound, right on the banks of the

Bendigo River or whatever it's called. Gum trees and mozzies on the glinty water. Stuff that Buddhists love. Like no grog or drugs. Hadn't counted on that. Or all the vego food.

'I've been here two years and three months,' the monk said. 'Why?'

'You ask the wrong questions.' 'What is this? Karate Kid?' He laughed again.

'You Karate Kid!'

'It was self defence!'

The monk kept grinning.

'You end up in prison, if not careful. Why so angry?'

Oh, Jesus, I thought. I know why. And I don't care. Angry Dad, angry brothers, angry life. Copped a few, whacked a few others. Who gives a shit?

'Okay, I'll calm down.' 'What if I do this?'

He dug his fingernails into the bare skin of my thigh below my shorts. I grabbed his hand and pulled it away.

'That fucking hurt!' 'It was supposed to.' 'Not very Buddhist!' 'What if I do this?'

I got ready this time. But he just stroked my knee with his skinny brown fingers.

'Get off!' I grabbed his hand and threw it back at him. 'Which worse? Pinch or stroke?'

'They were both shit.'

He stared at me and I watched the river. I listened to it trickle and carry on. A bird flew along the water like a fighter plane. The gums smelt like cough lollys. I looked back at the monk and he was still gawking at me and grinning.

'That's a bit wrong, all that staring . . .' 'Gay?'

'God, no! I don't care about gay! My brother's gay. I think. I just don't like being looked at for ages. No matter if you're a woman, a bloke or a fucking ox . . .'

'The ox . . . He is sacred animal. You are size of ox!' He laughed again. Like an idiot.

'Can we go back to base now?' 'You are uncomfortable?'

'No, I'm fucken bored.'

'Only boring people get bored.' 'Well, I'm boring then. Let's go back.'

It was afternoon meditation and snack coming up. Chill out time then vegie rolls.

'We go back,' the monk said, 'but not so angry.'

We sat in a circle on a huge mat with our eyes closed. We hummed. I could still feel the monk's hand on my leg. I opened my eyes. It was still there all right, the pressure of it, but no hand. Just something throbbing for a second under my skin. And then it was gone.

Three months in a monastery is a long time and it gets into your head. I didn't come out Buddhist or anything, but I was different. Not talking in riddles like they did, just thinking different. I still trod on ants, but only if they were annoying me outdoors with the students. And I thanked the ants in my head beforehand. For doing what they'd done in the circle of whatever.

It got worse at work rather than better though. I mean, I was doing my job well, I was caring for the kids, but a seventeen-year-old girl with black dyed hair decided I was so nice she wanted to have sex with me.

She talked to me after a metal work class and there it was, her hand on my knee. Her short skirt riding high up her leg till it was more than leg. I freaked. And ran.

Bosses got pissed off with me again.

'Doc, we can't have you running away from students. They've had people deserting them all their lives.'

'She wanted to get it on!'

The bosses, one male, one female, both in fashion combat shirts, laughed at me.

'Don't kid yourself, Doc,' the woman said.

I jogged all the way down to the Maribyrnong that night. I hadn't been to the factory for weeks. I had a bout coming up though and I thought a decent run and some of my old practice wouldn't hurt.

I went straight up to the shit-coloured wall, the little blobs staring at me, and I thought, Why the fuck did I ever do this? I started dancing and sparring, but I didn't throw any punches. I mean, who punches brick walls with their bare hands?

I did. And now I was chicken.

I watched the golden Buddha shining his arse off. I wondered why I hadn't thought of it before. Because gold is heavier than wall maybe?

I ran across the footbridge, through the reeds and into the Buddhist Temple grounds. No one came at me, but I could hear chanting and humming and all that business inside.

I went straight up to the golden Buddha boy and threw punches at him. He was hollow. He was made of some tinny shit and just painted gold. I belted into him and it sounded like thunder. The monks in their brown sacks walked out in a row and watched me for a bit. Then they laughed their bloody heads off and joined in with me until I was laughing so much I had to stop punching.

Fresh Dirt

Meg McNaught

Thumping wakes her. Pounding, on the door, not inside her head. Ella throws off the doona and stumbles out of bed. Knocks her toe on the door frame.

'Hello?' A voice from outside. More pounding.

Sliding, socks on hardwood floor. To the front door. She can make out the shape of a head through the wedge of glass. A woman's head. Ella swings the door open.

Fiftyish, dark suit, red lipstick. Lawyer? Uni lecturer? The woman looks Ella up and down.

Ella tugs at the sleeve of her hoodie.

'Good morning,' the woman says. She firms her lips. 'I just killed your dog.'

Ella squints. Early sun coming in between the trees, sneaking under the roof line.

'It ran in front of my car. I swerved, hard. But it kept coming. And I hit it. Here,' the woman opens her handbag, Prada the gold plate says. The woman is handing Ella money.

Ella doesn't move.

A crease runs between the woman's eyebrows deep enough to slice her face in two. The woman waves the money around, conduct- ing a symphony of sympathy in front of Ella's blank face. The woman sighs and presses the cash into the crook of Ella's elbow. 'I need to go.'

Out on the street, tyres screech. Ella looks past the woman and they watch a car veer around a lump in the road.

'I'm sorry,' the woman says and clips down the front steps in black heels. Ella thinks she used to have a similar pair. The woman gets into her car and slams the door. From the veranda Ella watches the woman drive away, wishes it was that easy. To just drive away.

'Hello, love.'

Ella turns. On the footpath stands an older gentleman. Ella has seen him before. On mornings when she has yet to go to bed – afraid of what lay behind her eyelids – sitting out here in the wicker chair, wrapped in an itchy blanket.

The older man is in shorts, despite the morning chill, and wears a neon headband. Tufts of his white hair poke up. 'Would you like help with your dog?'

Ella looks down at him, glances out at the lump in the street. Shrugs. As she steps back inside the fifty dollar note floats to the ground. Ella picks it up and closes the door. 'I don't have a dog.'

She trudges back to bed. Pulls the doona over her head. It isn't spring yet but she'd left the window open all night, cold air keeping her skin alive. She hears rustling around the rubbish bins beneath her window. 'This'll do,' a craggy voice. The man with the neon headband. He begins whistling. Ella follows the tune in her head Somewhere over the Rainbow and crimps her neck up trying to hear the last few notes as the melody fades. A few minutes later the whistling is back. More rustling, the plastic bin lid drops shut. Is he going to put the dog in the bin?

'No.' Ella shoots out of bed. 'Dead things do not go in bins.' The words snap around the empty room. Ella moves to the front door, down the steps and around to the side of the house.

The man is near the bins, stick legs poking out from his running shorts. 'Sorry about your dog, love. I didn't want to leave him lying there.'

Ella doesn't stop until she's right in front of him. 'Dead things should be safe.'

'Yes,' he says, watching her, in a way that is kinder than hospital staff.

'What are you doing?' She asks. 'With it. Him.'

'I found a box.' The man nods at the box sitting at his feet. 'He's a lovely chap. Gotta name?'

'Ella.'

'I thought he was a he?'

'Oh, right. Sorry.' Ella runs a hand through her hair and hits a knot. Damn. She turns her back to the man, pulls out her hair tie, smooths her hair back as best she can and swings it all into a pony tail. Her hair is dark so he won't be able to tell it hasn't been washed since. Since when. She has no idea. She turns back to him and clears her throat. 'Thank you for your help.'

'No worries at all love.' His eyes warm. 'I'm Fred. I'll do the digging.' Ella glances at his arms, skin flapping like wings. 'I can manage.' He hefts the box. 'Let's manage together.'

The only thing she's managed in the past two weeks is to breathe. And make tea. So much tea she is sure it flows milky grey through every vein in her body. This inept, lacking body that let her down. Let everyone down.

At the back of the house is a small garden with one big poinciana tree. Ella stops and looks around.

Fred puts the box down. 'I reckon here could be tricky,' he points to the base of the tree where large fingers of root grip the ground. 'How 'bout the back corner, behind that shrub.'

'Okay.'

'I'll need a shovel.'

'Of course.' Ella returns to the house, an old Queenslander, raised, the underneath closed in with slats of wood. She opens a gate- like door and walks in, the air cool and earthy. She has never been under here; she's housesitting. Soon she has to be ready to go to her own home. To walk into her house and up the stairs and past the room with the white crib that will remain empty for the foreseeable future. Jason is there. She misses him, would like to lay her head on his chest and listen to his beating, broken heart. But facing him, his green eyes soft with tears. Not yet.

An assortment of gardening tools lean against the wall. She grabs a shovel and a mattock – she'd seen her dad use one when clearing a patch for veggies. Fred is sitting on the back steps, tying an expensive running shoe. She sits down on the step below him. He hands her a blue collar. It's new. Two tags: one yellow plastic with numbers, the other metal and in the shape of a paw-print, Rusty. She turns the tag over. A phone number. Somewhere, someone is waiting for Rusty to come home for breakfast.

Ring the number.

And say what to Rusty's parents? Something pathetic. I'm sorry for your loss.

Her doctors were matter of fact. 'Miscarriages happen all the time.'

Not to her. To them. Jason had cried. Ran his hands through his hair and walked from the bed to the window and back a hundred times. When he reached for her, she curled away. Couldn't be touched. Her heart dangling by a cord.

Fred is pushing himself off the step with those wiry legs and walking toward the back fence. 'I'll start digging. Go ahead and have a few minutes with your fella.'

On the outside of the box is a picture of a microwave, the owners must have recently bought a new one. Ella wouldn't know, she's been eating straight from the tin. She imagines a dingo-like dog with reddish fur squished inside, forming a circle, so its head is touching its tail. Ella runs her hand over her stomach. Tears press. She holds them back, purses her lips. Heat swells inside her, a flush flames her cheeks, sweat trickles between her breasts. She yanks at her hoodie then flings it over her head and tosses it to the ground. Chilly air nips her bare arms.

Ella swallows. She breathes through her nose, kneels on the grass and lifts the lid of the box just enough to slide the collar in. No sound when the collar hits fur. 'I hope you had a good life, Rusty.' She closes the cardboard flap but keeps her hand on the box for a moment.

They'd called him Nick. Nicholas Ryan Moore. After he'd died they gave her nothing to hold or to wrap in a fuzzy blanket or put into a box. Ella had raised her head and watched a nurse leave with a yellow bag. 'Hey,' she called, 'Bring that back. My baby's in that bag.' Her shoul- ders were pushed onto the table. A mask pressed over her face. When she woke, Jason was there. His tie hanging as lopsided as he looked. After he kissed her forehead and walked away in the dim hospital light, Ella asked two different nurses where they took the babies, the ones in yellow bags. The first nurse suggested she try to sleep. The second offered her a drink of water. Ella swatted the glass away. 'I don't want fucking water. I want my baby.'

Fred is whistling again. Let's go Fly a Kite. Ella remembers watching the movie, Mary Poppins and that last scene in the park; the whole Banks family together, complete.

'Do you have a dog, Fred?' The way he presses his foot onto the shovel and scoops dirt, Ella can tell he's done this before.

'Grew up with them, lived closer to the bush then. Too crowded in the city to be having a dog if you ask me.' He turns and nods at the microwave box. 'Truth in point.'

'Yeah.'

He swipes at his mouth. Looks at the box, looks at her. 'How bout you get me a cold drink?'

Ella goes up the back steps, realizes the door is locked and makes her way around to the front of the house. She has kept herself to the spare bedroom, the veranda and the kitchen. A plate is in the sink with a mug although she doesn't remember eating. She flicks on the kettle. If she was at home, cold filtered water would be in the fridge. Jason always makes sure the pitcher is full. She fills two glasses with tap water and takes them out back.

Fred is scooping dirt and throwing it into the hole. The microwave box is nowhere to be seen. Gone. Just like that. Rusty's body, probably still warm, stashed away, covered with dirt. Eventually daisies will be planted. Or something. For seventeen weeks Ella carried her baby in her uterus, where he lived and where he died. One moment her body was sustaining him, keeping him warm and safe and fed; he was sung to and talked to and patted and photographed. He showered with her, went to work, nestled on her lap while she was driving. At night, when she and Jason were hugging, she felt the baby move between them.

'Love? I'm done here. Let's sit a spell.'

On the steps again, Fred leans back on both elbows, gazes up at the poinciana tree. The limbs bare and skeletal. Too early for nubs of green.

'Not an easy way to start the day. You gonna be okay?'

'I'll be fine.' Ella picks at a crusty stain on her track suit pants. She will change her clothes today. She will shower and comb her hair and put on something that fits. And she will ring Jason.

'Time I finish my walk, then.' Fred gets to his feet.

Ella stands, too. 'This was very kind of you Fred, to help me.' She feels tears building again, lowers her voice to a whisper. 'Why did you help me?'

He reaches out and squeezes her arm. 'It's what we do.'

Ella nods, watches him go. The morning air is warming. Around her, the smell of the fresh dirt lingers.

G

Roland Leach

He woke to what may have been an animal sound and sensed she was outside the window. He jumped out of bed and leaned into the darkness, seeing her staring up at him, not saying a word. 'I'll be three minutes, I'll grab some apples.' They walked down the hill and saw the back reefs breaking like white flowers against a darkness that was just shifting beyond that moment where the edge between night and day tips to a soft shadowless visibility. Then walked along the coast road to the Point, their boards beneath their arms appearing in the darkness as either weapons or celestial wings.

They had been going down the beach together every day during the holidays since they met. He was hand-fishing on the reef when he noticed a girl coming down the sandhill. He turned back, concen- trating on the tension of the line, lifting it slightly so it went taut, so any nibble would be noticed. Then she was there, only two steps away from him, already preoccupied with her bait being fixed securely and focusing solely on the water below her.

They didn't speak and even when she caught a fish and Roald congratulated her she ignored him. When leaving, he said goodbye and began walking up the sandhill. Near the top he realized she was behind him, walking slowly now, though she must have run up the hill to have been so close. They crossed the coast road side by side and walked up his street, until at his house he turned and told her he was going in for lunch.

She spoke for the first time. It didn't sound like a fourteen year old's voice. More like a voice that had been fermented for years in a barrel or maybe a well, sounding as if it came from a distant place.

'You live 'ere?'

'We moved in last week.' 'What you doin'?'

'Just having lunch.' 'You comin' out after?' 'I suppose.'

'I'll come back and wait outside for you.'

That had been six weeks ago and they had been inseparable though she didn't talk very often and he knew almost nothing about her. She came to meet him every day. When the surf was on the rise she would go to his back window before dawn so they could get to the Point before the crowd. Other days she would sit and wait on the front verge and they would go to the beach and body surf or fish or roam the bush north of where the road ended.

There had been only three days when they had not spent their days together. G stayed with her uncle on occasions, she didn't say why, but said it was always for three days. He would pick her up and take her home with him.

It was just at the end of these three days, during the middle of the night that Roald heard a skateboard, the clunking roll of tiny hard wheels on asphalt, and knew it was G. His room didn't face the road but he stuck his head out the window to try to hear her. The moon was almost full and he could see it tangled in their jacaranda in the back yard.

Next morning G was sitting on the verge. She had a skateboard and he could see she was proud of her new acquisition. She held it up as if she were presenting it formally to him. 'Look. My uncle gave it to me.'

Roald liked the idea that G was an anonymous being who had suddenly appeared like a mythical sprite without parents, a proper name or home, though he knew she lived only a half-mile away but the skate- board and the existence of an uncle made G, the girl with an initial as a name, connected to a more prosaic world.

The skateboard was not new and was a little battered but he said it was great. 'I heard you go down the hill last night.'

'Did you? I wanted you to. It was almost a full moon.' It came out fast and staccato. She did something then that she had never done. She raised her chin and pretended to be a wolf and made a low howling sound that made Roald think of dark forests in fairytales, but then it shifted to what sounded like the purring of a great cat. She had never been not her, never acted or spoke without being prompted. She was always G: quiet, unanimated, never joking, without irony or artifice. Now she seemed play acting.

'Do your parents let you out in the middle of the night?' 'They're dead asleep.'

The first thing Roald's Mum said when she saw G was that she looked like a street urchin. That hair of hers, and what was she wearing.

G was tall for her age, skinny, suntanned and had sun-bleached straw for hair. Roald had not noticed at first but her clothes did look worn out. They were faded as if all the colour had been washed away.

On their way home from the Point they would stop at the shop over- looking the bay. G would roll cigarettes – she carried an old packet of Drum, the plastic cover almost worn away, which she refilled each week by stealing from her Mum's pack - and Roald would buy a carton of milk and choc milk and they'd sit at the stool table and look out to Rottnest. Then they would walk home on the path that ran along the ocean, saying little and always an arm's distance between them. He didn't know what that space meant but it was there: along the coast road, on the beach, through bush tracks, it was there.

One day looking out at Rottnest, after a day at the Point, G started speaking.'We went to Rottnest. Me and my mum and dad and my brother. I was coming down a big hill with my brother on the front of the bike. I peddled as hard as I could, then I put my feet on the handlebar.' She drew back on her cigarette. Roald heard the inhala- tion of breath, the small sigh.

'We come off. I scrapped all the back of my legs and bum. My brother hit his head on the road. It was sharp bitch'men. The blood was all over it.

G had never spoken so many words at one time. She was staring out at Rottnest, the island a mirage of grey castles and cliffs. Roald didn't know if he should say anything, then asked how long ago was the accident.

'I was ten and my brother was eight.'

When it came out, the event turned into words, it seemed to Roald that G appeared surprised, as though she had never said it before and now spoken was different to the thing she remembered in her head – that block of wood, the black sludge – that she had been carrying for nearly four years. She shrugged her shoulders and went back to looking out at the ocean, then lit another rollie and gave it to him.

A moment later she said she couldn't have a bike now, and then in another voice, not her own, she muttered lowly, 'That will teach you for killing my son.'

'What did you say?'

'Nothin'.

He was thinking about G's brother when his Mum came into the kitchen and hugged him.

'Have you been smoking? Has that girl given you cigarettes?' She was a woman who didn't wait to hear answers she already knew. 'I heard from Marguerite who just lives over the hill and a few houses up from your girlfriend.'

'She's not my girlfriend', Roald intercepted, hoping to turn the subject away from him smoking.

'Well your friend then, the one you spend every day with from dawn to dusk. She said that the family is a wreck. Her mother spends most of her day in bed on tranquillizers. Drinking coffee and smoking cigarettes.' She stopped and looked her son in the eyes. 'And the father is a real no-hoper. Never worked a hard day in his life, has tattoos all the way up his arms, and heaven knows where else and is a heavy drinker.'

She also wanted to mention how the girl roams the street at night and that there is no one at home to control her, no school in her life, and just too much freedom for a girl her age. Marguerite told her G had a 'history'. But she decided that was for another time.

Towards the end of the holidays Roald and G stopped at Mick's, his best friend who had been in Ireland with his family. Roald threw his board on the lawn and went to the front door while G walked up the long gradient of street with her skateboard. Mick came out from the beneath the house where he had been playing table tennis and called to Roald.

Mick was telling him how he had missed out on summer and Ireland was fucking freezing, before his older brother appeared. Greg never uttered a sentence without its sole purpose being an insult or a laugh. He was usually laughing as he said it, and only stayed for as long as it took to deliver his lines. He laughed out the line, 'priests and nuns everywhere. Mum and Dad had a fucking ball. Thought it the last stop before heaven.'

Just then G came down the street on her skateboard. Greg watched her flick her skateboard into her hand and said, 'Well who's this, then?'

'She's a friend,' Roald said too loudly.

'Roald find himself a girlfriend over the holiday, while the compe- tition was out of town.'

'Get lost.'

'Mind that language, young man', Greg laughed out.

'Must be a real summer romance if you get so heat up . . . ' He stopped and looked at G. 'Hey, is that the girl who gave Mark . . . ' Before he had the word out Roald ran straight at him and gave him a hip and shoulder to the chest. He had no inkling that he would ever do that off the football field but for a second he was standing there with the older boy flat on his back having trouble breathing. As Roald and G walked away he heard Greg spluttering, 'You little mad shit; fuck you and take your mole.'

They didn't say anything till they were nearly home and Roald asked why she never talked about her parents. She didn't reply but sort of shrugged.

Roald tried again. 'If you had to use one word to describe your Mum what would it be?

'Sad.'

'And your Dad?' 'He's a cunt.'

She wasn't on the verge the next day. When she didn't turn up the following day Roald walked over the hill and went to her house. It wasn't quite as bad as he expected so he walked up the stairs and knocked. The woman who appeared looked young but as Roald observed her she seemed to grow older.

'Excuse me, I am a friend of G. I was wondering if she was home.'

G's mother was wearing an old cardigan though it was a hot morning.

'I'm sorry' she said, and Roald really thought she meant it. 'She's staying with her uncle.'

'When will she return, if you don't mind me asking?'

'I don't know'. Pausing before she continued, 'I don't know', and walked away without closing the door.

When Roald returned three days later there was no one home and it felt like a house abandoned.

It was almost the end of the holidays though there was a good month of summer left. The following day there was an unseasonal storm, the remnants of a dying cyclone that had trekked south but had turned out to sea and had lost strength.

Blackberries

Jessica Clements

She dreams of blackberries and wakes with the memory of sweetness on her tongue.

She hears the baby cry but when she opens her eyes the room is silent and the light around her dim. Mild summer wind drifts in through the window and brushes against her arms, exposed from the thin cover of the cotton sheet her husband is still cocooned in. The baby is asleep beside her, unmoved from where she had placed him in the pram what seems like moments ago but is probably more like hours. She reaches over and presses a finger underneath the shadow of his button nose to feel the tiny stream of breath pulsing out. It is one of the many habits she has acquired over the past four months that would sound maternal had she heard them from anyone else, but to her they are nothing more than routine. The last time her husband caught her doing this he smiled and said what a good mother she was, and she felt like a fraud. She pictured his face if she told him the dreams she'd been having, or the thoughts about her once wished for child.

She looks over at her husband in the bed, face down and breath- ing heavily into the pillow. In a couple more hours he will have left for his office in town and she will be alone again. During the days there is no one for company but the baby and the neighbour's horse; a beautiful bay-coloured gelding who sticks his head over the fence when she is in the garden and blow lips as if he disapproves of her.

She slides out of the covers and wheels her sleeping son carefully out of the bedroom and through the house, stopping to slip on the thongs that lay beside the back door. She pushes the pram down the slope of their property – not quite big enough to be called a farm save for a few chickens and a vegie patch. She is careful and focused as she walks and only has two things on her mind. In one step she silently pleads with the baby, don't wake up. On the other step she pleads with herself, don't let go. It would be so easy, she thinks in the calm of the early morning, to let go.

At the bottom of the hill she stops the pram and squeezes on the brakes with her foot. She pulls the empty bluebell bowl from the basket below her sleeping boy and sits down on the cool dry grass. She faces the bushes speckled with fruit that have formed a wild green tangle alongside the drying creek, and reaches up to pluck a berry from the stem, dropping it into the bowl.

Taking the journey to the edge of the garden in the early hours is another routine she's developed in new-motherhood. Already she must've picked half the fruit off the bush; the laundry floor encum- bered with buckets of berries, stewing as they sit beside the warmth of the dryer. Her husband calls the bushes weeds and tears them down each year with an axe. But when she looks at them she sees childhood summers at her grandmother's house in England, where blackber- ries lined every road and twisting country lane. She sees giant silver pots boiling on the stove and dozens of steaming glass jars overflow- ing with warm, sticky fruit. She's tried to remember her grandmoth- er's recipe but her jam has never quite turned out the same, always coming out sickly-sweet and runny as egg white. She wishes there had been a cookbook among the items her mother had sent her after her grandmother had died. A glass rabbit heavily padded in bubble wrap, a handmade quilt, and few mismatched teacups and chipped mixing bowls were all that had been saved.

She traces the pattern of blue flowers along the chipped edge with her thumb, feeling her eyelids grow heavy again. When her doctor first suggested taking up a hobby, she stared at him blankly, wondering for a moment if he was the one who had gone temporarily mad.

'What kind of things did you like to do before?' he asked her. 'Any hobbies? I hear knitting is big these days . . . ' She was just glad he didn't mention mothers' group. The thought of a bunch of women sitting around at the park discussing whose baby could turn himself over already was enough to make the familiar churn of morning sickness rise again in her throat.

'Branch out,' he told her, 'don't be afraid to try something new'.

Her husband pointed out that he didn't think the doctor had meant for her to take the advice so literally. But at least she was getting out, even if it was just to the end of their yard, and only at night. Picking blackberries is the only thing that calms her. It gives her something to focus on in between feeds when she feels the walls of the house folding in on her and all she wants to do is escape. Her doctor called it post-na- tal, but whatever it was it had been there once or twice before. She recognised it like an odd scent she couldn't place or a flavour that had slipped from the tip of her tongue. The only difference was that now she had the baby, and he had to come first no matter what she felt. The problem was, what she felt wasn't always easy to push away.

The baby stirs and lets out a wail. She jiggles the pram with her free hand, hoping he will go back to sleep.

Sleep. How long has she been out here? She looks up and sees the sky paling into gradual daylight. She leans back on the grass. Even with her eyes closed she still sees blackberries. She dreams about them too sometimes. She sees their branches reaching out towards the pram and wrapping their twig hands around mottled pink baby legs, holding onto them like unripened fruit. She can almost feel the baby rising in her arms and then pushing him into the prickly bush, further and further, until something inside her snaps.

Her husband calls her name from the back door of the house.

The sky has lightened quickly. Morning again.

She brings the fretting baby away from the sharp branches and places him carefully in his pram, walking back up the slope of their yard to where her husband waits for her with a coffee in hand. When she gets inside she thinks, they will have breakfast together and she will feed her son. They will listen to him make small noises of hungry desperation that will make them both want to laugh. She will say to her husband that when the baby is old enough, maybe they could take him to England. He will smile and tell her that she could make jam, and it will come flooding back to her in a rush, the smell of blackberries and fresh lemon. Sweetness with a hint of sour.

Jupiter Rising

Dorothy Simmons

She smiles, reaches across the bed for him.

Not there. No steady breathing, no grizzled chest hair. Gone. She must start wearing pyjamas.

News radio. The oldest person in the world is 117. That's 57 years older than her. 55 years older than Jack. Would have been.

Her phone rings. Tom probably, twins still sick, is she OK to babysit again?

No. School. She'd forgotten about school; it's not on her radar any more. Though she's on theirs, apparently, or at least their relief teacher list. Never took her name off, did she? Well, fuck that. Not what she needs.

But she just heard herself say yes. What is she thinking? Call back, apologize, sorry Mary, automatic pilot . . . except it's not Mary, it's somebody new. Mary would never have called her.

They must be desperate, phoning this late.

She hasn't seen anyone from school since the funeral. She closes her eyes, visualising the walk from sign in book to staffroom, scanning all the sympathetic faces. The classroom: benches, sinks, trays, bunsen burners: you in the back row, take those things out of your ears . . . no. Can't. Can't. Cancel.

But her finger hesitates, hovers above her phone. Take her name off that list, and that's it. End of that story too. Along with the papers signed, the handshake with the new owner, the keys to the new apartment. From the bedroom window, she can see a corner of the new owner's Kenworth. Beside it, their caravan is a dinky toy. Yet only three months ago, poring over maps of Australia, they'd worried in case it was bigger than they needed.

They probably are desperate. Not many relief teachers about, not in Science, and definitely not in the country. Rare bird, hey Jilly? The Lesser Rural Casual? There's always been as much work as she wanted; she'd had a desk in the Science staffroom for years. So why not? What else is she going to do? Walk the dogs. Pack. Clear his office instead of walking in to it and straight back out again. Practise for the weekend scattering of his ashes. Practise reading his poem, though she could never do it like him: On a starred night Prince Lucifer uprose . . . who'll climb their hill and recite poetry now?

She puts down her phone and swings her legs over the edge of the bed. Dammit, take her mind off things. They won't get anybody else, not this late. And there's still their last payment on the caravan. Correction: her last payment. Before she sells the damn thing.

So far so good. Juniors: couple of budding smart arses, couple of mummy's little hand wavers, lot of ordinary kids paying ordinary attention. No different. Why would it be? Only three months, not three years. Class dismissed.

In the Ladies, the big mirror hangs exactly where it's hung since that first day she walked in and stuck out her tongue at her probation- ary self. How many years ago? Miss Miller: big hair, suede waistcoat with fringes. She sighs. Mrs. Lawson: cropped white hair, cardigan.

The door slams. A swirl of glossy black hair, hands grabbing the basin, shoulders heaving as she retches: Jill rushes over, grabs paper towels, turns a tap on.

In the mirror, long dark eyes meet hers. Must be new; they get younger all the time. Asian, by the looks. Wiping her mouth, the young woman draws herself upright.

'Thank you. Sorry. ' Her eyes register the white hair, the cardigan. 'Sorry to scare you.'

'Nonsense. You're not well. You need to lie down.'

'No, I'm OK. I am: just . . . something I ate. Like, last night. I feel better now.'

'You should have stayed home, you're in no state to teach.'

'I am, I just did: double Prac. HSC Science.' She raises a palm to June's protesting face.

'No, really. I will be fine, don't worry.'

'Well, is there somebody I can call? Come on, let's at least get you to the staffroom '

'The common room. It's closer: common room.'

They walk in silence. In the common room, they sit opposite each other, waiting.

'Thank you. My name is Melissa. Melissa Chen. Are you a teacher?

I have not seen you before.'

'Jill Lawson. Sit down, I'll get you a glass of water.' Keep talking. 'I'm actually a Science teacher here too, though I haven't worked for a while. You haven't been here long? No? Thought so. I only do relief work now. Mind you, damned if I know who it's a relief for sometimes. I prefer 'Casual'. More '

'Laid back.' Melissa takes the glass and smiles. 'I am Casual too. In place of Mr. Barnes: he had a car accident.'

Jill nods; yes, of course, Greg: she should have been to see him.

'You're taking his classes then?'

'This term. After that, who knows? I hope there will be more work'

'Well, Greg was supposed to retire last year. So you're in with a chance.'

'Really?' Melissa's face lit up. 'I came down from Sydney for this job. I have been trying to impress Mr Carver . . . '

Good luck with that. Dan Carver: Head of Science. Head bean counter. Also due to retire; not before time.

'But he is . . . well, he is '

'Set in his ways.' Not to say one-eyed, dogmatic. 'I suppose he's asked where you're from? What you're doing here?'

'Yes.' The nod is vehement. 'I told him to mind his business.' 'Uh-oh. That won't have gone down well.'

'No. I should have bitten my tongue.'

'What about the kids? How are you managing with them?'

'The kids are OK.' A dismissive wave of the hand, a wince. 'Most of them. Most of the time.'

'That'd be right. Once they get to know you, they're usually OK. You be straight with them, they'll be straight with you. Or that's what I've found. As for Dan Carver, just keep doing your job. Sticks and stones, you know.'

'Sticks and stones?'

'Old saying: sticks and stones may break my bones, but words will never hurt me.'

'Stupid saying.'

Yes. Yes.

In the darkened classroom, Tom Hanks hurtles across the universe. Apollo 13: reward for improved behaviour, reads the note on her lesson plan. And because it's last period Friday, thinks June, hovering behind the fidgeters and nudgers in the back row. It is a really old film; the digital natives are restless.

'Why's it called Apollo 13, Miss? Isn't 13 unlucky?' She pauses the movie.

'Apollo was the god of the sun. Back before science started, that's how people explained what they saw around them: the sun, the moon, the sky, how day turned into night. They figured light must travel, and because they travelled by chariot, and because light came from fire, they figured the sun must be a fiery chariot, drawn by fiery horses. And the driver must be some kind of superhuman, a god: Apollo. For the moon, they had a goddess: Diana. Day, night: sunshine, moonshine.'

'Hey . . . Dinah's my name, Miss!' The girl in the back row flares mascara hedged eyes.

Jill shrugs and nods. 'Well, there you go. You're a goddess!

'See my streaks?' Dinah fans fingers through her hair. 'Moon Silver, they're called.'

'Who cares? Press play, Miss, get to the bit where the oxygen blows up.'

'Yeah, Clarkey, all that hot air!'

'Did they really believe all that crap, Miss?'

'Would we believe in blood cells if scientists hadn't seen them through a microscope? The ancient Greeks only had their naked eyes.' 'Woo hoo, naked eyes!'

‘Dinah’s eyes aren’t naked but they’re covered in fly shit!’ ‘Fuck you, Clarkey!’

The text book spins through the air, clips the boy’s eyebrow. He jumps up, yelling and bleeding. Dinah stabs her finger upward. ‘Effin’ little smartarse!’

‘Stop! Cut it right there, you two!’

June slams the car door, leans back. Apologies all round, if they’d known, of course . . . hope she got the flowers. Yes, thank you, thank you…never sent a thank you note . . .

Jack would have laughed. Made her see the funny side: lights up, he’d say, come on, lights up. Fly shit for make-up: he’d have liked that. Made some crack about black humour, walked her up the hill, *it seemed the best thing to be up and go . . . .*

She turns the key in the ignition.

Message from Tom: all set for tomorrow. She glances at the photo of Jack with the littlies and bites her lip.

OK: office. Walk in, sit down. Where to start? Accounts, Weekly Times, folders, papers: Astronomical Society flier. Special event: unique opportunity to see Jupiter rising. That’s right; they were going to go. Biggest planet in the solar system, Jilly, right up close and regional! He’s circled the date. It’s at the Wetlands, where they go birdwatch- ing. Went birdwatching. She looks at the date and catches her breath.

Tonight. She looks at her watch.

The Wetlands car park looks different at night, eucalypts spectral against a darkness seeded with tiny spores of light, billions upon billions of them . . . light years of them . . . .

Jack’s friend Clive coughs and says how sorry he is. She mutters about finding the flier. Somebody calls for him; he’s the Club Pres- ident now. He pats her shoulder, leads her to a telescope, urges her to take a look.

Pressing her face to the viewer, one eye squeezed shut, the other squinting up and down and around, she can’t see a thing. Jack would have seen it straight off, of course. Smartarse. She stands back, shaking her head. Try again. Up close and   there, suddenly there,

is the moon. Like in the magazines, craters and that   what, some

kind of cosmic Rorschach Test? No: the Sea of Tranquillity, that’s what it is. Come forth into the light of things   so many quotes, how

did you remember them all?

But where’s Jupiter? Jack? Where in God’s name is Jupiter?

She still hasn’t found him when they are summonsed into the Wetlands shed. Its walls have been painted: emu, platypus, wombat. There is a poster headed ‘Under Wiradjuri Skies’. Clive is talking: something about a website.

Someone touches her arm.

'Melissa! What on earth . . . I mean sky'

'Ha! I'm a member. This is Zac, he works here'

The young man beside her grins and nods. She smiles at Melissa. 'You OK now?

'Yep, I'm fine. Lights up.' She leans her head against the sun on Zac's T shirt.'When will you be in again?'

'No idea. Hadn't planned on being in again at all.'

'What? But why not? I was going to organize an excursion. Out here. Local area, local flora and fauna. I was going to ask for you as the second teacher'

'Good idea: thanks. But Dan'll probably insist on someone permanent.'

'But you said you've taught there for years, that you might as well be permanent. He'd be OK with you, surely'

'Well: maybe. Tell you what, tell him you got the idea from Greg.

In his files or something: it's the kind of thing he would do.'

'Listen everybody!' Behind them, Clive coughs and taps his watch. 'Jupiter, OK? Time!'

'Jupiter schtupider. Can't see him for the life of me.'

'What? Can't see the Lord of the Rings?' Zac takes Jill by the arm. 'Come on!'

'Lord of the Rings? Isn't that Saturn?'

'Yeah, him too. Grumpy old men. Come on.' Jill hesitates, then lets them bustle her out.

'Over here,' Zac points. 'Now, get the angle right '

Amazing things, telescopes. How they can make the whole universe… local.

A nudge from Zac. 'Found him yet? Found the rings?'

'No, too stupid. Keep losing myself; no, wait there! Yes!'

In among all the billions of microcosmic spores, flung through time and space with his reckless lassos of dust dust we are, as dust

we're reborn Jupiter shines.

On a starred night Prince Lucifer uprose . . . .

Not Lucifer, Jack. Jupiter rising.

Quotes:
'On a starred night Prince Lucifer uprose.' - Lucifer in Starlight, George Meredith
'It seemed the best thing to be up and go.' - Aubade, William Empson
'Come forth into the light of things' - The Tables Turned, William Wordsworth

Animalia

William Stanforth

'Who gives a fuck if the polar ice caps melt?' Ian said, hunched forward in the dark room, pulling his socks on. 'Why does it matter?' Kate released the blind and the grey autumn light flooded in.

Harsh shapes filled the room: a vintage dresser from hard rubbish, a queen-sized bed pushed into the corner, clothes strewn everywhere. She looked out the window and into the front yard. She said, 'Those old Italians are taking our olives.'

'I said they could yesterday,' Ian found his glasses on the bedside table. 'But seriously, who cares about climate change, bees dying at an unprecedented rate, humanity's looming extinction? We're looking at these problems the wrong way. We should be deciding if we're worth saving in the first place. Weighing up the odds, you know? Because we could be wasting our time.'

'Please don't make this a big deal,' Kate said. 'I thought you'd find it funny. I did.' She was referring to a series of Instagram direct messages she'd shown him in bed moments earlier. The messages came from a stranger in the U.S., and they were mostly just photos of the man's penis in various stages of erection, and one of him coming. There was also a text that read: Id love to kno wat u taste like baby.

Kate had not replied.

'It's not that I don't find it funny,' Ian said. 'It just makes it pretty hard to reconcile with other people, seeing those photos. Think of all these Hollywood films, someone's got the nuclear codes, a comet's hurtling towards Earth, and we must find a way to prevail. But why? Why are we worth saving?'

'Look,' Kate said. 'I didn't mean to upset you. This isn't a threat to you. It's not like I'm gonna see something like that and think: wow, a random dick . . . god, I wish I could fuck it. And jeez, predatory messages really get me going.'

'I know,' Ian said, sighing. 'It's not your fault.'

'How could it possibly be my fault?' Kate asked. She turned the oil heater off and started making the bed, 'So I can't share photos online? I've gotta censor myself living day to day? Besides, you're in at least half of them.' She smiled, 'Maybe he thinks he's talking to you.'

Ian stood up and started rifling through the dresser. 'Don't make this about you. I'm not angry or jealous . . . it's deeper than that.'

Kate said, 'What do you mean?'

'I mean there's gotta be a certain number of reasons to keep persisting in life. And when some fuckwit sends photos of his genitals to you, and I think about how the images probably bounced off satel- lites or under the pacific to get here, it just throws the whole balance out.'

Kate moved back to the bedroom window. She watched the older couple outside, 'Did you say they could take all of them?'

Ian said, 'We can't just be animals, you know?'

'Well imagine how I feel?' Kate said. 'I have to deal with this all the time.'

Ian pulled on a woollen jumper and grabbed his keys and wallet from the dresser. 'What do you mean? How many dick pics have you received?'

Kate said, 'Like the total number of photos? Or men? Is that what you're asking?'

It was difficult to tell if the elderly couple outside were arguing or just having a fervent Italian conversation. The woman steadied a ladder as her husband balanced precariously and shook the branches. The olives fell into a green net on the ground and the old man noticed the younger couple, then descended the ladder.

'Thank you,' he said, switching to English. 'We'll come back for more later.'

'No problem,' Ian said, opening the small gate for Kate and then walking out into the street. The wind sent a sharp chill through the air as they wandered towards the supermarket. Dark storm clouds rolled overhead and Ian wrapped his jacket around his body and leant into the wind. The weather seemed to awaken something in Kate. She twisted around a parking sign and pretended to dance with it for a moment. She said, 'What do you feel like for lunch? I'll make you anything you want, baby.'

'I don't care, what do you think?' Ian said. He couldn't get the images out of his mind: a bowl of soup, a baguette, and then there it was, creeping into the frame, throbbing and coming. The man's face did not appear in the photos, but Ian could see someone: thirty-some- thing, receding hairline, muscular, solarium-tanned, walking around some modern, tasteless apartment in grey track pants, watching a massive flat screen television, scrolling through images of Kate, touching himself, coming.

Ian shuddered; he realised he hated this man as much as he could another. He then looked at Kate; she was running her hand along the rusted wire fence of a local school, composed, smiling faintly. For a moment, he resented her beauty. He wished he'd fallen for someone less attractive, plainer, someone who didn't draw the attention of random men online. And then he resented himself.

There were about ten homeless people at the supermarket entrance. Most of them were men and two were in wheelchairs. Half were drinking cheap cider from brown plastic bottles, and one sat cross-legged with an empty bottle crushed in his hand, body tilted forward, head almost touching the pavement.

Ian had walked past them many times before, and when he first moved into the neighbourhood he'd sometimes give them a little spare change—though he'd since stopped doing this and didn't know why. Now they were part of the scenery: living effigies with spider veins and broken capillaries. One would leave or die and some poor soul would take his place, for reasons no one likes to think about.

Inside, there was the usual Sunday afternoon rush: families with screaming children, young professionals preparing for the week ahead, searching and grabbing under the low, fluorescent sky. A group of teens were buying cask wine at the adjacent bottle shop, kicking on from a big night. One of them, a young girl with dark brown hair, held a bottle of orange juice, and Ian felt suddenly nostalgic. Kate said, 'I kind of feel like paella.'

'That sounds nice,' Ian said.

'And you can take some to work tomorrow.'

'That sounds nice,' he said again. He watched her pick out the vegetables and put them into a basket: red and yellow peppers, chillies, an onion, some garlic. He followed her around the store like a small child, studying her movements. She collected the rest of the ingredients and a few things they needed at home. She picked out the most expensive coffee, and Ian said, 'I don't get paid until Thursday.'

Kate said, 'Don't worry about it.'

At the self-serve checkout, she turned the coffee's barcode away from the scanner and bagged it as potatoes. She placed a bunch of other items on the scale, chocolate, shampoo, toothpaste, and scanned them all as brown onions. She weighed the actual vegetables and payed the balance with her credit card.

'Aren't you scared they'll track you down?' Ian said.

'And what will they do?' Kate asked. 'I'll say I thought I was using it correctly. Can they prove I have any idea what's going on?'

They walked outside and rain started to pour out of the thick, charcoal sky. The homeless people had already dispersed, found shelter some- where nearby. Kate and Ian stood under the awning of a small café and watched as the sidewalk flooded.

Kate said, 'Let's wait it out.' Ian nodded and they went inside and sat by the window. The waitress came over and took their order, just coffee. Ian was silent for a while and when he looked at Kate he realised he was trying to smile.

'Don't you find it distressing?' he said. 'Aren't you worried you'll be standing next to someone like that at work or on a train?'

'You're not still thinking about that, are you?' Kate said.

'But doesn't it make you dislike men? Dislike me? What do you think it means?'

'Nah,' she said. 'And I don't think it means anything, other than that particular guy is a creep. That's all. Life's a lot more enjoyable when you lower your expectations of other people, especially the people you don't know.'

Ian said, 'Yeah, I guess.'

They sat in silence for a moment and the waitress arrived with their order. Kate stirred sugar into her coffee and asked, 'Aren't there enough good things to keep you persisting, as you said? Aren't I one of those things?'

'Yeah,' Ian said. 'I was just being dramatic. I was getting protective. I'm sorry. I'll let it go.' He wanted to tell her the kind of influence she had, the power of it, but feared it would change things, come across as needy. Eventually the rain stopped and the storm clouds started to clear. They paid the bill and walked out into the street. The homeless people were settling back in at the supermarket's entrance, emerging from the shadows of some dark recess or god knows where.

When they arrived back home, Ian washed the dishes and Kate turned the radio on. A world news update was broadcasting and a man with a British accent spoke of a landslide in Nepal, a tectonic plate shifting, thousands presumed dead. He reported on a young man who'd entered a Turkish airport with explosives, nails and screws strapped to his chest. The man detonated the device, the journalist said, sending shrapnel outwards and into the unsuspecting living.

Kate then scanned the airwaves for another station, 'The horror of the daily news,' she said, 'lies in the details… it's knowing the size and weight of an average screw, of a nail.' She stopped on a station playing some old modal jazz, Miles Davis or other, trumpets pulsating through the heated kitchen air, bouncing off the chipped walls.

Ian was still thinking about the Instagram messages, though he could feel himself moving on, his anger fading. Part of existing is forgetting, he thought. He found himself visualising the teens from the bottle shop, wondering what they were doing: probably sitting in a park, drinking cheap wine, not yet burdened by adulthood's growing pressures. In the vision, Ian saw the young brunette girl smiling right at him, the only face in the faceless.

He'd quit smoking months earlier, but he had the sudden urge for a cigarette. In the bedroom, he found an old pack he'd been hiding deep in a dresser draw. He grabbed a box of matches from the kitchen table and headed outside.

The afternoon light was fading and the elderly couple were back and almost done at the olive tree. They were now in yellow rain- coats and gumboots and the woman held a large multi-coloured umbrella. Ian watched them for a moment and then looked out into the street. He sensed a kind of violence in the atmosphere, an uncer- tainty down the bluestone alleyways and on the tenement rooftops – behind the apartment doors and in the cars driving slowly on the soaked bitumen.

The ladder was around the other side of the tree and the old man straddled the top rung. He shook a distant branch as the woman steadied it and looked up at him.

'Scimmia, scimmia' the woman said, grinning.

They both turned from the tree and noticed Ian standing on the porch.

Ian lit a cigarette. 'What's that?' he said. 'What does that mean?' The elderly woman said, 'How do you say, ape? Like a monkey?'

Her husband imitated, with his thumbs in his armpits, then hitting the last olives from the tree.

'He's an ape,' the woman said laughing, eyes closed, keeling forward, barely able to keep the ladder still.

Look Me In the Eye

Sophia Barnes

We didn't know until the next day that the old man had been killed. We kept playing for hours in the dry heat, the astringent smell of eucalyptus mixing with sandstone dust in our nostrils. The creek had slowed to a trickle a few days earlier so now there was only damp mud, pockmarked by the jagged rocks we threw down the slope and into the trees, as hard and fast as we could.

When we grew tired of that we wrestled, chasing and falling in the scratchy undergrowth. Ants in their universe of labour moved beneath and around and over us, across splayed arms and grazed knees, unfazed by our violence.

I read this back just now and at first I didn't notice it. When I say the old man had been killed, he is the subject: he has met with misfortune. If I say we killed the old man, we are the subject, and he is the object. We are the misfortune.

My mother had begun to make dinner when we came home; I could smell the onion cooking from the back gate. She used to buy those TV guide magazines with the recipes on the back page: Four simple meals for your family! Six ways to cook cauliflower! I helped her sometimes, chopping ingredients, measuring out water for the rice. It comes in handy now that I live alone.

In the kitchen the old metal of the stove cracked with heat from the grill. A clove of garlic had been left on the cutting board, and a greasy knife lay on the table by the door. She must have been holding it when she heard my father talking to the neighbours, and carried it as far as the door before she realised.

John and I were covered head to toe in the dark orange dirt from the creek bed, my knees bleeding and he sporting an ugly bruise on his cheek where I had hit him. We didn't see the neighbours until we had gone all the way through the house, following the noise of voices.

John edged forward onto the porch to eavesdrop, keeping out of my father's sight until we'd had time to wash. I stood on my tiptoes to see over his shoulder.

'No time to save him, too much blood,' Mr Jessup shook his head, frowned, pursed his lips. I remember him looking the same way the day he came to tell us that wildfires had taken out half of Tarella, up the highway. I think he liked being the bearer of bad news.

My mother had a hand up to cover her mouth, still clutching a tea towel like she was shielding herself from a bad smell, or holding herself back from throwing up. Mrs Jessup wasn't there and at first I didn't see the others – Mr Coleton and his son Michael, who had just finished school. He was old enough to stand with the adults, while we hid behind the railing.

'Cut right into his skull, you could see the bone showing—' Mr Jessup stopped and looked at my mother, unsure. 'Pardon, Kate, I'm only repeating . . .' he trailed off.

My father seemed to remember something then, and he took my mother's arm, so that the tea-towel pulled away from her face.

'Katie, you should check on the boys.'

I think my mother was annoyed, but she didn't argue. She turned away from the men and came up the stairs till she was looking right at us.

'Boys! What are you doing out here? Go on, get back inside,' she pushed us in through the door and part way down the hall. 'Out the back, under the hose, get that mud off.'

Normally we would have caught it worse for coming inside like we were, trailing dirt, with the blood from my cut knee trickling down my calf and onto the rug.

We washed in silence, turning the hose on each other and kicking our feet under the nozzle. John didn't mention Mr Jessup or the Coletons so neither did I. When we came into the kitchen only three plates were set. My sister was staying the night at a friend's house, and my father had gone out.

'They need him over at Mr Caffey's, but he'll be back soon,' my mother said. I looked at John to see if he would ask why, but he was silent, so I didn't ask either. I didn't often speak unless John had spoken first.

The next day my mother wore her outside clothes inside. A few men from up the street sat in our front room, looking uncomfortable, their terse conversations punctuated by long stretches of frowning silence.

Cara came home and locked the door to her room. She didn't talk to us anymore now she went to high school, she just spent all day on the phone to her boyfriend. Sometimes John and I would sneak into the hall and pick up the extension, making silly noises into the handset until she came running out shouting at us to piss off. We couldn't do it, though, with all those neighbours around.

My mother told us to stay near the house, so we climbed up the elm tree by the back toilet and shot seeds down at the corrugated roof. No one used it anymore but it still stood, weather-beaten and leaky, with a solitary half-used roll hanging from the hinge inside.

At lunchtime we followed our empty stomachs into the kitchen. There was a tray of sandwich triangles sitting on the dining table, thick with cheese and slices of tomato, red juice slowly leaking into the bread. We picked up four or five each, stuffing the first into our mouths in one bite. John leered at me, wet crusts squeezing out either side of his teeth, and I stuck my tongue out in response, spitting crumbs onto the floor. I didn't notice my mother come in.

'What are you doing? Stop mucking around.' She reached out for John's arm and saw the mess squashed in his palm. 'Those aren't for you! Two each, that's it. Put that back.'

She picked up the tray. 'Go back outside,' she said, and went into the living room to feed the men.

We walked to the edge of the garden, where the old wire fence sagged under the weight of blackberry grown wild. John kicked at the ground, making rough dirt holes in the patchy grass, restless. We weren't used to being kept this close.

John dared me to climb over the fence and run down to the creek and back. A dare from John could usually persuade me to do almost anything, but I shrugged him off. The year before he'd dared me to steal Cara's diary, a thick exercise book laminated and embossed with stickers she collected from music and film magazines. She yelled and threatened for a whole weekend but John wouldn't tell her where it was. Finally she cried, and I gave in.

We didn't even open it up, and now I don't think that we would have understood anything in it if we had, but John knew that taking it would upset her. When I handed it back to her he didn't talk to me for three days. Then I got into a fight with Jamie Coleton before school and John joined in, giving him a sweltering bruise that he had to hide from the teacher for the rest of the day. After that he seemed to forget that he was angry with me, and things went back to normal.

Children don't think of the months in the same way adults do—they live by changes in the weather, the shortening of afternoons by the creek or on the street; the leaves of the tree next to the back toilet changing colour; whether it's hot enough to run under the sprinkler in shorts. So Mr Caffey died before the summer storms came, when the heat was fierce but not heavy, and the eucalyptus leaves broke into tiny pieces under your feet.

After the neighbours had cleared out that day, our mother let us back inside. She sat us down at the dining room table, though it was an hour at least till dinner time. As she spoke she looked from one of us to the other and back again, anxious to see that we understood.

It was a rock that did it, right in the back of the head. He'd been out picking up rubbish along the western edge of the creek, the other side from our house. We saw him doing that sometimes, collecting the beer bottles and chip packets that kids from the high school left down there. I didn't see him, but I reckon John did. He told me he'd hit a magpie – said he'd heard the squawk as it fell. We never went to check.

A few days later my parents drove us into town and left us at the cinema with money for a movie and some popcorn. I suppose they were going to the funeral. Mr Caffey had lived on our street all my life, so all those neighbour men would have gone along too.

School started again a week later – I was going into grade five, John grade six. No one else's parents had told them much more than my mother had told us, but Jamie Coleton said he'd heard his dad and Michael talking about it. Jamie held onto the story like it was a packet of lollies, doling out the details one by one, enjoying the notoriety.

'His head was smashed open,' He told a pack of us at recess, eyes wide.

'A big rock,' he whispered loudly to a pair of girls in math class. 'Blood everywhere. Dad said he didn't have a chance.'

I woke up screaming, that night or the next, although I don't remember the dream. I know that my mother came in to calm me down. John and I slept in the same room, me on the bottom bunk and he on the top.

My mother and father were talking about it the next morning, before breakfast; I heard them from the hallway outside the kitchen. John came up behind me and stood quiet, waiting.

'But we have to tell someone, don't we?'

There was silence for a little while before my father replied, his voice low.

'What good would it do?'

I heard my mother sigh, the way she did sometimes when she thought she was alone.

'He might have killed someone, we have to—' 'No one knows that. Just let it go.'

I could hear my father moving towards the hall, so I stepped forward into the kitchen, keeping my eyes on the ground. He paused for a moment in front of us then walked quickly to the front door, slamming it closed behind him.

John and I didn't play together as much after that summer. He started hanging out with the other year six boys at lunch, while I sat alone on a bench down the back of the oval. After school he played soccer in the council park and on the weekends he would go into town to the shopping centre. No one went down to the creek anymore after Mr Caffey died.

The next year John went into high school, and after that he disap- peared. At first it was only in the afternoons until dinner, then some- times overnight, but by the time he started year nine it was for days at a time. He went for good when I was fifteen, and I haven't seen him since. The police told my parents that they shouldn't assume the worst: sometimes kids do that, just up and head off, and then they turn up, months or years later, perfectly safe. It's been three decades now though, and I don't think John is coming back.

Blue Day

Beverley Lello

I summon my daughters to spend the weekend with me at our beach house. 'Just us,' I say. 'No husbands, no boyfriends, no babies.'

I spend an hour alone in the house and stumble over Harvey's presence everywhere: his shaving gear in the bathroom, the copy of Dispatches from Syria, half-read on the bedside table, his battered beach hat hanging on the hook at the back door. He's even caught in the cobwebs draping the outside windows, there because I'd asked him to climb the ladder and brush them away and, like so many jobs, it was something he'd get around to doing when we retired and came more often.

The rooms are trapped behind closed doors, smelling like decades of damp towels and salty shell collections. I open windows then wander onto the deck. From here, you can see the dunes, smooth hillocks of white sand. Beyond them, through the late summer haze, lies a vast expanse of indigo ocean, the horizon a ruled line separat- ing it from a pastel sky. A blue day, we used to call it. Today, I would prefer it to be grey.

On the beach, visible from the deck, there's a single red-and- white umbrella flapping in the breeze, a scattering of sunbathers and two small children building a sandcastle. The season is nearly over and nobody has been to the house all summer.

Keira arrives first, gives me a quick kiss and a hug. 'The waves are perfect,' she says. 'Not to be wasted. Come to the beach when Franny arrives.'

She'll drive her van, her home since Harvey died, to the car park closer to the surf beach. He attempted to teach us all to surf, but Keira was the only one who persisted through the dumps and tumbles. They shared the same determination to be very good at everything they tried. Was she still trying to prove to him that she could be the best?

When Francesca appears, she sighs, kicks off her sandals and says, 'I should come here more often,' before slumping into her favourite deck chair, thumbs already tapping at her mobile.

'Zac,' she says. 'You'd think he'd know by now that Rose needs to be put down for a nap mid-morning. I've been gone three hours and he's feeling trapped.'

While I wait for her to finish texting, I scatter seed for the rainbow lorikeets, letting them know we're back. It's a feeding frenzy.

Husks fly; blue heads bob and sideways eyes peer from a gleam of green feathers. Feeding the birds was always the first thing Harvey did when we arrived at the house. If I squint, I can see him holding out the Arnott's biscuit tin with the picture of the horse and cart, with Frances- ca, when she was small, cupping the seed in her hand to lure the birds to settle on her arm. She's squealing at the pricking claws but standing fast as they peck from her palm.

Francesca finally looks at me. 'You shouldn't feed them,' she says. 'They become dependent.'

'They seem to survive when we're not here.' I sound defensive. She stops tapping. 'Are you mad at me?'

I'd usually say, 'No, no. Not at all,' but if I did she might keep texting, forcing me to stand up, grab the phone and hurl it into the air. The lorikeets would take flight. So, all I say is, 'It would be nice to talk.'

'I'm a teacher, Mum. I have a baby. And it was a long drive.'

I ram the lid back on the seed tin and hold it against my chest. More gently, she says, 'It's about Dad, isn't it?'

Harvey's heart stopped beating one morning, somewhere between his cereal and his toast and coffee. The toast, slightly burnt on the edges, remained in the toaster until I returned to the house later that night. I remember thinking from then on there'd only be one slice.

Harvey and I were on the edge of doing all those things that pepper conversations in the last months of full-time work. We'll cycle in France. Spend weeks, not weekends, at the beach house. Read more. Now, I didn't want to do any of those things.

The beach house, a fibro hand-me-down from his own parents, was our haven when the girls were young. It was our escape from the city, a place where sandy feet inside were tolerated, meals tossed together and housework only done when we packed up to go home. When Harvey was here, he'd be mowing the grass, or sanding back the wind-scoured west wall and adding a new coat of paint, or heading to the beach with his surfboard.

It's not a haven anymore, just another reminder that I'm on my own. I've decided to sell it because my heart aches when I think of coming here. The girls, I know, will not be happy, but I tell myself they've stayed away too. Even good memories can cause pain.

Francesca puts the phone to one side. I have her attention now. 'Everyone keeps telling me I have to move on,' I say. More words

bubble out. 'I used to wake up and think of all the things I wanted to do. Now I see the day as a vast hole to be filled in.'

The phone pings, but she ignores it. 'I'm sorry, Mum. I miss him too.' She struggles out of the deck chair. 'It wasn't supposed to be like this.'

'Oh, Mum.' We hug. How much I miss someone holding me. 'You've got a lorikeet answering your text message,' I say as we separate.

The birds have eaten all the seed, but a loner is pecking at Franc- esca's mobile as if this might be the source of more. She snatches it up and the bird flies off to join its flock in the scribbly gum next to the deck.

'It's Keira,' she says. 'Wants us to meet her on the beach. To show off, I suppose.'

I'll tell them I'm selling when we get back. I can't keep hanging on to the old life, I'll say.

We walk along the shore. The surface of the ocean sparkles like the sequins I once sewed onto the girl's dance costumes. The waves inflate into languid humps, arch and spill into a cascade of froth. On the sand, translucent blue jellyfish litter the high tide mark, their stinger tails like kite strings pointing toward the abandoning ocean. Their presence reinforces that surface beauty can be deceptive; a seemingly healthy body can harbour a faulty heart.

'No way I'd swim today,' Francesca says, popping one of the puff bags with her sandalled foot. I think of the lorikeets on her arm. Not always so cautious.

Closer to the rocks, Keira is knee-deep in foam, clutching her surfboard, looking as lithe in shape as the wave that curls toward her. She spots us, raises her arm then thrusts the board into the wave and paddles out beyond the break.

We dutifully watch her catch a wave, wobble, but hold her stance. She paddles out again. Doesn't even make it to standing on her next attempt. Topples. Surfaces. One arm clutches the end of the board before she loses her grip when a wave crashes over her and sucks her under again. The surfboard, freed, rides a wave toward the shore. Keira rises from the foam, utters a yelp of pain and claws at her shoulder.

'Stingers,' Francesca says smugly.

Another breaking wave topples Keira and she struggles to stand. Francesca wades in and grabs hold of the ankle strap on the surf- board and drags it onto the dry sand.

Keira lurches toward us through the shallows. 'It hurts.' 'A stinger. They're all along the beach,' I say.

'It's like red hot needles.' 'Vinegar.'

'It's in the food box in the back of the van. Shit, it hurts.'

She ploughs across the sand and up the rickety steps to the car park, Francesca and me in her wake.

The back of the van is a fug of smells: damp towel, unwashed socks and pizza. It's also a chaos of clothes, take-away containers and empty soft drink bottles. I rummage in a box of food supplies. The plastic bottle of vinegar is buried under several cans of baked beans. My itin- erant daughter, adrift without her father to anchor her down.

I grab the bottle and a T-shirt and upend the vinegar onto the soft fabric. I dab at the long red welt. The tension in her body ebbs. I'm reminded of grazed knees and bumped heads; I feel needed.

'Thanks,' she says. 'A dramatic homecoming.'

'Your grand entrance, again.' Francesca laughs a little. 'It's still stinging, but not so much.'

I shake out the T-shirt and notice the Quiksilver logo. 'Sorry about my choice of a rag.'

'It needs a wash.' She smiles, rupturing a crack in her lower lip. 'Your surfing's improving,' says Francesca generously.

'Not my best effort.'

'Dad would be pleased someone in the family's keeping it up.' Keira is silent. She reaches out and squeezes Francesca's hand and

I'm happy to see my girls connect.

Francesca breaks the spell. 'Hey, maybe we could all have a few days in the house at Easter. It's time Aunty Keira got to spend some time with Rose.'

'Only if I don't have to babysit,' she says.

Keira slips the T-shirt over her head, fixes me with her sea-blue eyes and says, 'The house, Mum. We need to talk.'

Francesca glances at the van. 'I'll walk home.' 'You could sit in the back,' Keira offers.

Francesca wrinkles her nose, looks at Keira, then me. 'I need the exercise.'

I sense a conspiracy. They know I've summoned them for a reason.

Francesca strides away; she seems to have her energy back.

I shift a pizza box onto the floor of the van and climb into the passenger seat. I feel young and ridiculous sitting here, the smell of vinegar on my fingers and salt on my skin. It's like stepping back in time, Harvey at the wheel of the old VW Kombi, the surfboards roped on the roof; then, years later, with the girls, buckets and spades and

boogie boards in the back of the Holden station wagon.

Keira climbs in and we sit in a companionable silence, looking out to sea. My decision hovers, but I'm feeling less convinced that it's the right one.

'I was wondering,' she says, 'if I could live here for a while. I want to go back next semester and finish the Film and Television course. I'll work in the bakery. Save some money.'

At the mention of the bakery, I immediately think of Harvey's love of fresh bread rolls on Saturday mornings, before realising that Keira wants to live in the beach house. I could come and not be alone. Maybe, Francesca would occasionally join us with Zac and Rose. White light shimmers on the surface of the indigo sea. The waves keep tumbling, frothing up onto the sand. The blue day that seemed so wrong is starting to seem right.

Francesca beats us back to the house. I see her on the balcony, seed in the palm of her hand, the lorikeets balanced like acrobats along her outstretched arm. She calls out, 'Look, Mum. Look!'

A Bad Friend

Emily Riches

Ted had always been a doggish person. Not only did he resemble one—so wiry and thin you could see every bone in his body—but he followed you around like one too. He leant on you. He was always nervously twining his arms together and clasping his hands: thus contorted, they looked awkward and inhuman, like forelegs. In this way, he drew attention, without meaning to, to the small pale scars laddered there. He had golden skin and hair that began high up on his forehead like an old man's. Even when we were younger his voice was deep and sarcastic, almost gravelly, as though he was speaking through a perpetual chest cold. He had dark eyes, more pupil than iris, and long sensitive lashes that curled so far up they smudged his glasses.

In school, I was always worried that people would think he was in love with me, or that he actually was. This made me feel both powerful and embarrassed, and determined whether on a given day I was friendly or cruel to him.

For instance, one morning I spotted him pacing back and forth in front of the school gates, scowling. I knew he'd be waiting for me: he'd called me all weekend and I'd ignored all his messages, rolling my eyes each time with my friend Freya. Before he could see me, I ducked down to the oval where my friends gathered before the bell. We laughed about my narrow escape.

Yet soon they saw him walking across the grass towards us. 'Hide me!' I cried, and was immediately buried under an avalanche of schoolbags. I lay as still as I could, breathing heavily, heart thudding. My friends arranged themselves nonchalantly over the pile.

'He's coming over,' Freya hissed. 'Be quiet Moira. Ok, he's stopped. He's looking, still looking . . . Don't move! Alright, he's leaving. He's gone. You can come out.'

'Did he see me?' I gasped. 'Probably. He looked sad.'

I had no classes with Ted that day but slunk around school, spending lunchtime buried behind a Stephen King novel in the library, watching him drift past the tinted windows like a lost dog.

He intercepted me at the buses when the final bell rang. 'Where have you been?' he asked, his lip pushed out. 'I called you all weekend. You didn't answer.'

'I was busy,' I lied queasily. 'Family stuff.'

I knew he didn't believe me but I couldn't think of anything else to say. I looked around to make sure someone like Freya hadn't seen us. He drew a short snuffling breath as though about to cry and thrust one ankle out at such a sickly angle that I felt ill and found myself touching his shoulder, apologising, promising to come to his house that afternoon. He looked at me so deeply with his wet grateful eyes that I almost shuddered.

Weeks later at my eighteenth birthday party, I watched Freya kissing the boy I'd been in love with for the past year. Ted sat down next to me, too close. 'It's ok,' he said, slinging his bony elbow over my quaking shoulders. 'It's ok.' We'd both been drinking. The room swayed. I shut my eyes and leaned against him for a moment as he hugged me sloppily, breathing into my neck.

'I'm fine,' I said, shaking him off, hoping no one was looking. Later, at one a.m. we danced crazily together, holding hands and spinning, both out of breath, collapsing on the lawn. I let him sleep on my bedroom floor that night as Freya and I shared my bed, our foreheads pressed together, my heart breaking.

On the last day of school, Ted and I skipped class together and walked into town. It began drizzling rain and unsure what to do, we slipped into a café. He was nervous at the counter, waited for me to order and then ordered the same. We sat at a table for two, self-conscious as though it was a date. Our conversation was strained, neither of us wanting to admit the afternoon was already a failure. I was abrupt and unforthcoming as he hunched over his cappuccino, looking up at me through his eyelashes. He stirred sugar after sugar into his cup.

'I don't really like coffee,' he admitted.

'Why did you get one then?' I asked, incredulous, and he shrugged, smiling weakly. His lips were wet with foam.

'So, are you and Freya talking yet?'

I glanced at him, put down my cup. 'We're not not talking.'

He looked cowed. 'Sorry. I just meant, after the party and everything.'

'Oh.' I forced a loud laugh, brushing it aside. 'That was nothing. She's my best friend.' The words slipped out of me like a wraith, silvery and juvenile.

Eventually, I walked him part-way back to school to catch the bus, joking and happier now that the date was over. Each time our shoul- ders bumped together I felt a rush of warmth for him. We parted with a bony sexless hug and said 'See ya later,' like kids in an American movie. I walked back home along the main road, glancing up each time a bus drove by. When I saw Ted, he was sitting backwards in his seat, looking for me. We locked eyes; he smiled, lifted a hand. I didn't wave back.

We both ended up in Melbourne after high school, living a few suburbs apart. I was staying with my grandparents while I studied, and Ted moved into a dingy one bedroom flat, waiting tables at night. We saw one another a lot in the beginning, both of us lonely and overwhelmed in this new city.

I wasn't sure how it happened exactly, but slowly our interactions became more formal. My grandparents invited him to Sunday lunch. We went out for dinner in a fancy restaurant and both fumbled to pay. Once, he snuck a bottle of wine into a violent action movie but neither of us were confident enough to drink it.

I normally walked back to his house after these dates. We talked on his couch, our knees touching until the unspoken expectation of sex made me panic and find an excuse to leave. One night, however, I lingered until I'd missed the last bus. We were sitting side by side watching a movie when he rested his head on my shoulder.

His voice was soft. 'Will you stay?'

I didn't say anything. The urgent, pressing need of him. I shook my head.

'Why not?' he pleaded. 'I just can't.'

'Moira . . .' he whined, at such a pitch that I leapt up and yelled, 'Why can't we just be friends?'

Ted was shocked. He sat with his hands on his knees like a person awaiting death by the electric chair. His eyes were glassy, his lips parted. I stood up, flushed and embarrassed at my outburst, but he didn't move, even while I gathered my things and left, feeling sick and cowardly.

Our friendship never recovered. For a time, I was the one leaving messages, fervent apologies soaked in guilt, while he doggedly avoided my calls until I gave up and we didn't speak for almost two years. I studied hard and didn't date much. When I did, I attracted men like him: needy and nervous with big beautiful eyes and thin sickly wrists. We'd go out for dinner at expensive restaurants, each time ordering lots, eating little. Later, they'd kiss me at my grandparent's front door, pressing me against the wall until the weight of their expectations sickened me and I pushed them away. They'd call again the next day, hurt but persistent, and we'd try again until finally they got fed up and stopped calling. I'd wait for them to text me, weep when they didn't, and then retreat—relieved, defeated—back into life alone.

Then, a classmate's wedding in August: a mutual friend, Brian from high school, was marrying his long term boyfriend. Our whole year was invited and a group of friends were flying in from Brisbane, staying in a hotel together. I saw Ted from a distance at the reception, hanging at the fringes, his hair longer, a wine glass clutched in his hand. For most of the party, I sat with my old friends in the cloakroom, smoking cigarettes and cackling. Whenever anyone walked in we hid behind piles of coats, giggling like mad, crying 'Mr Tumnus, is that you?'

Freya blew smoke through pursed lips: 'Ted looks different doesn't he? Remember that time in high school when he ran away from home and caught the train all the way here?'

I stared at her. 'What? I didn't know about that.'

'He had problems, you know? I heard he talked to people on the internet and came down to meet up with one of them.' She gave me a smug, chilly stare.

'That's wild,' I said. 'What 'people'?'

Someone else shrugged. 'Maybe it was a boy? I always thought he was in the closet, not like Brian. Hard to meet people in a small country town I guess.'

'I thought he had a crush on you Moira. He idolised you. Remember how he used to follow you around?' They all turned to stare at me, grinning.

'Yeah but we were just friends.' I felt strange and bitter towards Freya for bringing it all up. I drifted out into the party, grimacing at people I did and didn't recognise. I contemplated slinking out, but couldn't face rescuing my coat from the cloakroom. I quickly found myself at the bar and ordered a shot in case I had to walk home without it.

'Moira.' It was Ted. He looked sunken around the eyes, almost bruised, emaciated as a model. We hugged stiffly, then went into the foyer together, to sit and drink and talk. He worked as a bartender now, stringy muscles clinging to his arms. He had a small fashionable moustache and strong cologne. It was hard not to keep looking over my shoulder for Freya.

'Are you seeing anyone?' he asked. I said no.

We weaved back to his house, arms linked. I felt warm, forgiven. Pleasure bubbled up in my chest like a kettle. He still lived in the same flat, slightly less bare but just as dingy. I was surprised we hadn't bumped into one another the last two years, but didn't say it. He poured me another drink and trained his eyes on me as I wandered around the room, picking up books from his shelves.

'Hey listen,' he said, 'I'm getting rid of most of this stuff soon. So if there's anything you want, you can have it.'

'Bit of spring cleaning?'

He took a sip of his drink and swallowed. 'I'm moving, actually.' 'Oh?' I felt gracious and cheerful, like a good friend. 'Do you

need a hand?'

'No, thanks. Should be fine. I'm leaving next week.' 'Where you off to then?'

'London.'

'Huh.' I breathed in. 'How long for?' 'For good, hopefully.'

I said nothing. Something was plummeting inside me, making it hard to speak, to stand upright. He was talking, asking about my grandparents and how they were doing but I cleared my throat, mumbled something and slipped into the bathroom. I crouched over the sink, drooling and dizzy with loss.

He knocked after a while. 'You ok?'

I splashed my face under the cold tap and called, 'I'm fine.'

When I emerged, I told him I wasn't feeling well. He offered to call me a taxi or to walk me home but I refused, fending off his kindness. I saw something wobble then harden in his eyes, some- thing that allowed him to shrug, open another beer, let me leave for the last time.

I lay awake all night. In the morning, dog tired, I called him but he didn't pick up.

Lucky

Alexandra O'Sullivan

The middle aged man across the counter is waiting for me to speak. He's wearing a white coat that's so clean it's hurting my eyes. My voice comes out too high.

'I'd just like the . . .' I drop it down a semi-tone, 'morning after pill, please.'

I watch his reaction. They always have a reaction, a slight widening of the eyes at the very least. Sometimes the eyebrows go up. He has his reaction, quite minimal as they go, then he scurries away from the counter to have a whispered conversation with his colleague, a short woman who is also dressed in a crisp, white coat. Her eyes flick to me, then back to him. Then she says.

'This way, Miss.'

I follow her to the far counter and try not to think about the meaning of her emphasis.

What's on tonight Miss? That's what Tom wrote to me last night. I looked at the text and felt a flicker between my legs. Miss. He only calls me that when he wants to see me. When he is able to see me. We hadn't spoken in a while. I also hadn't had sex in a while, though not for lack of offers. It's called 'getting lucky.' People say, 'Did you get lucky?' when they want to know if you had sex. Sometimes they say, 'Did you get any?' or 'Did you get some?' But it all means the same thing. Luck. Did you have any luck in the sexual roulette wheel otherwise known as 'dating' Only luck to me is not about whether you get it or not, but how good it is. That's the tricky thing.

I'm on Tinder, but I fucking hate it. There is no end to it, you could swipe forever. The faces blur together. On a date last week, I suddenly realised I couldn't remember if this was the doctor or the accountant or neither. It didn't matter. He was boring, whoever he was. No doubt he liked a quiet night in and the occasional night out. They all say that on their profiles, as if they're telling you a secret. I should put on my profile - I like to go inside and I like to go outside and sometimes I stand in the doorway and have an existential crisis. I think I'm having a sexistential crisis. I've been having it since

I last saw Tom. That was the night I got too drunk to perform. You wouldn't think that could happen to a woman, but it can. At least, if the guy is decent enough not to fuck a comatose starfish. And Tom is. Decent enough, that is. He's not decent enough not to cheat on his girlfriend, but hey, you can't have it all. I try not to think about her anyway. She's like Santa or God—an idea that doesn't quite come off in reality. But sometimes that makes her seem bigger, like she expands beyond my own earthly selfish desires. She doesn't need like I do. She's 'The Girlfriend.' She gets the whole biscuit and I'm the one scavenging around for crumbs. Maybe that's why I drank, that last time, to give myself a little more of a treat. But of course, that backfired on me and all I got was a hangover.

So, when he messaged me again I was excited. I zoomed around my unit tidying up, and tried several 'at home lounging around' outfits on in front of my mirror. It's more difficult when they are coming over to your place, not only do you have to get the right casual look, but when you're going out, eventually you just have to commit and leave the house in whatever you're wearing last. Whereas when you're staying in you can change and change and change back again, until they knock on the door and surprise you in your underwear.

At the last minute I decided to trim my pubic hair with the kitchen scissors, the same ones I use to chop basil and parsley. I couldn't decide how much to take away. I probably should have shaved it all because that's what's expected, but I'm no longer comfortable having sex with a newly scraped pubic area. It makes me feel skinned, vulnerable. What felt right at 21, now at 35 feels slightly ridiculous. So, instead I chopped carefully, keeping the blades tilted away from the little nub in the centre, wincing at the thought of slicing into that cluster of nerve endings. I threw the handful of wiry curls into the kitchen bin with the potato peel and tea bags, then scraped my hand over my newly mown Velcro-like crotch, easier to run my fingers through, more difficult to grab. I hitched up my underwear and jeans, poured myself a glass of wine, lit up a smoke and waited.

I'm hungover as I fill out the form at the chemist. When did the incident occur? Did the form really just use the word incident? I write in a shaky hand: last night. I don't know the date, I can't think well enough to work it out. Nausea hits me as I hunch over the form, I take a deep breath to hold it away. When was your last period? How the fuck do I know, I can't even remember what date yesterday was. When I woke up this morning, all I wanted to do was stay in bed, hugging at the cool side of the pillow next to me. I considered doing just that all day, and not bothering to get the pill, but that would have been irresponsible.

Now, as I scrawl my signature at the bottom of the form I think, what are the odds? What am I insuring against here? The very slim chance that it is one of the two days a month that I have an egg just sitting there ready for implantation, and that his sperm survived the long, treacherous journey through my body past all my internal defences and is now poised and ready to spear itself into this egg at any moment? It all seems so implausible. Nothing to do with him ever sticks. How unlucky would I have to be?

Last night, he stood in my kitchen leaning one hand against the counter top and holding a beer with the other hand. His shirt was slightly unbuttoned, like a hero in a Mills and Boon. My eyes were drawn to the deep V made by the fabric, to the smooth rounds of his pecs just visible, to the heart beneath. Was it pounding like mine? He drained his beer and looked around, then stooped towards the gap under my sink and said, 'Is this the bin?'

'Yeah.' I moved forward quickly to take the beer bottle from him and we grazed fingers. Zap. Like touching an electric fence, only good. I put the bottle in the bin on top of the scraps and curly hairs and turned back to him. It was one seamless move, an invitation from his point of view. And mine. We melted together. I thought about his girlfriend and melted into him some more. Transgression is so sexy. There was no going back from there. He floated me to my bedroom. I want to say we made love, although I don't know if I can quite claim that.

'Would you like some water?' The chemist's assistant asks me as she hands me the little packet. I see the chemist hovering behind, watching.

So I can take the pill in front of them and their crisp white coats and their staring eyes?

'No thanks.' I fork out $30 for the pill and head back to my car where I know I have a bottle of water. My hangover is really pressing down on me as I unlock the car and pull open the door. Inside it's hot. I take a sip from the stale water, then I open my little packet, press the pill out and hold it between my thumb and forefinger. As I lift the pill to my mouth it jumps from my fingertips. I watch it sail through the air and land somewhere on the floor of my car. I say 'fuck' loudly.

I can see it when I hunch down on the pavement next to my open car door. It's wedged itself between the bottom of the seat and the metal runner that moves the seat backwards and forwards. I can only wiggle one finger into the space, the tip presses against the pill, but it doesn't stick as I pull it away. If I could jam the little fucker into my fingernail I could get it, but it just won't get in there. I'm picking up crumbs instead and I wipe them off my fingertip angrily. I can see a shrivelled French fry and I'm tempted to eat it. Nausea swirls around my guts and rises towards my throat. I lean the side of my head against the steering wheel. The horn blares.

I think, fuck this and stagger into the nearest café for eggs and coffee. I sit out the front to drink my coffee and smoke a cigarette, drawing in as much caffeine and nicotine possible, making my insides inhospitable. It's hostile territory, nothing can survive in there. Through my smoke haze I watch the people walking by, carrying shopping or drinking from environmentally unfriendly coffee cups. A man is being led down the street by a dog on a leash. I feel as if I'm watching a movie scene, and all these people are just extras shoved in to make up a crowd, they don't relate to the story at all.

I inhale more smoke and blow it out in front of me. I can't decide whether to go back to the chemist and fork out another $30 and face their stupid faces looking at me again. Maybe I want something to survive. A tiny seed could grow into something more. I would have to tell Tom, I'd play up my emotional turmoil a bit, score some points. It would serve him right, he's the one who's been sprinkling crumbs all this time. But how lucky would I have to be?

I get pulled over by a booze bus on the way home. I'm directed to the front of the line where I pull up by the traffic cone. I breathe my bad breath into the tube pushed in front of my face and wait nervously in my stinking car. I watch the copper gazing at the little white tube attached to his hand-held machine as he turns his body and takes a step away. I wonder what he's thinking, if there's a part of him hoping I blow over, if that would give him satisfaction. Or maybe he wishes he never caught anyone drink driving. Maybe he has seen the heartache it leads to. The back of his head gives me no indication either way. He turns and comes slowly back to the window. He leans in. I hold my breath, his cheek is close to mine.

'Good result,' he says, and he waves me on with a smile.

Fantasia

Chris Flynn

My cocktail is going down a treat. Everyone else seems to be sippy sippy. I should really follow their lead. I have a bad habit of peaking too early. I need to learn how to pace myself, to not pass out and miss the main event. I must have watched the first two hours of Dances With Wolves five times. Never seen the ending. I assume hunky Kevin marries Kicking Bird and they spend the rest of their lives braiding each other's hair.

Ash reappears, a mischievous grin on her plate. 'What have you been up to?' Zoë asks.

She reveals a plastic Ziploc bag in her palm. 'Did you score some coke?' I say, unsurprised. Ash shakes her head. 'Nope. Fantasia.'

'What the fuck is that?' Phoebe asks. 'Dimethyltryptamine,' I tell her. I aced pharmacology at Uni.

'Dimethawhatnow?'

'DMT. Also called 45-minute psychosis. It's a dissociative hallu- cinogenic under which users allegedly share a communal experi- ence, in which they see vast alien landscapes and robotic elves, or something like that.'

Zoë and Ashlee's eyes turn huge. 'Holy fuck,' Ash says.

'Sounds friggen awesome,' Zoë adds.

'Yeah, I don't know about that,' I say. 'Where'd you get it, Ash?' 'Some guy. I wanted ecstasy, but he says this is way better. All the

cool kids are doing it.'

'Oh, well that's all right then,' Desley says. 'As long as the cool kids have rubber stamped it.'

'You don't have to take any,' Ash says.

'There's no fucken way I'm gunna.' She raises her cocktail glass. 'I'm sticking to good old fashioned liver failure, thank you very much.'

'Is Phoebe sleeping?' I ask.

Phoebe's head is lolling on Desley's shoulder. The booze has caught up with her. 'Come on then, who's going to do a line?' Ash shakes the baggy.

'I'm in,' Zoë says. Desley shakes her head. Phoebe is out for the count.

'What about you, Stel?'

Good question. Is this it? Is this the moment my life changes? I always knew there was a whole other world out there, and not even "out there" but in here, right here next to me, all around me, running parallel to my own but only glimpsed occasionally, always tantalisingly out of reach because I couldn't break through the wall, didn't hold the key, couldn't crack the password. It's more than the fear of missing out, it's the nagging feeling that I've been on the false path somehow, that I took a wrong turn when Danny first came in my hand eight years ago and I tried to discretely shake it off but ended up with jizz on my shoes, or maybe it was even earlier than that, maybe it was in High School when I stayed home to study after Evan practically begged me to come watch him do verts at the skate park. I should have been one of those girls who sat atop the ramp, Converse dangling as Evan rocketed up towards me and kicked, turned, flipped his deck and stretched his bony fingers out to touch my stockinged leg. That would have been a moment like this, an entry point to another life, a door opening. Or maybe I could have slipstreamed even earlier than that, when I was fourteen and Thuy said we should do it, we should jump from that rocky outcrop and plunge into the water of the bay but I was chicken, I was afraid of the current pulling me under and of getting my clothes wet and she went anyway, she leapt into the void and narrowly missed the rocks and I thought she was dead, that she would never come back up but she did and she shouted come on, Stel, do it, just jump but I didn't and when she showed me the huge bruise on her chest I was glad I'd been sensible but jealous too, envious of the battle scar she bore.

Could I have crossed over even earlier? When I was seven maybe, and we were up in Taree so Dad could watch his dumb powerboat racing and ogle girls with, "nice sets of lungs" and Mum wouldn't let me do anything, not even play soccer with the other kids because I was too frail and too smart and too gifted on the violin that I quit a year later, too destined for better things than organised sports. Could I have walked into the bush that day and disappeared forever, or at least until the disgruntled search party found me two days later? I wanted to. I wanted to run away and live with the wombats. I had Uncle Toby's muesli bars and a Sunnyboy. I had sturdy shoes. I had a dorky sun visor and a secret penknife my parents didn't know about.

But I didn't go. I held Mum's hand and watched Dad whooping as speedboats roared past, spraying the small crowd on the foreshore with a fine mist of crisp lake water.

This is one of those moments again, one of those potential turning points I have always shied away from. Instead of embracing possibility,

I have been imagining my life instead. Dreaming it, while I've been living it. I've always fantasized about another version of who I am, the brave, impulsive, reckless, adventurous me who gets lost in the bush and free-falls past sharp rocks and sticks my pointed tongue in the mouths of strangers. This whole time, I could have been a differ- ent person. I should have been a different person. Instead, I've been a cowardy-custard, a poltroon, a fraidy cat. And now, as a result, I'm a haunted thirty-two year old, a twitchy geyser about to erupt. I am Strokkur. I am Old Faithful. I am Beowawe. Whoosh.

'Fuck it,' I say. 'Line me up.'

Ash prises open the Ziploc bag and shakes a quantity of the powder onto the tabletop. She produces my MasterCard and divides the drug into three lines. Zoë is ready with a ten-dollar note, rolled into a tube. Gangsta. She hands it to me and I lean in, not hesitating for a second longer. The drug is bitter at the back of my throat and I have to swallow a long draught of water to mask the taste. Alien landscapes, they say. Let's give it a go. I shut my eyes and imagine myself living in a small habitation on some distant moon—Europa, Ganymede, Callisto, Io—looking out through a porthole at the bleak terrain. I am a first generation colonist, terraforming the landscape so others may follow, long after I'm dead. There will be a school named after me, maybe even a statue honouring my exploits as a brave explorer of the new frontier. Jupiter dominates the sky, its anti- cyclonic Great Red Spot a permanent storm, larger than our distant homeworld. It is silent but for the hum of machinery.

Strands of Jupiter

Rashida Murphy

Our resident astrologer was a strict vegetarian Hindu who wore his caste marks on his forehead. With stained fingers he spread out charts and filled the room with the smell of ink and cigarette smoke. His hands were papery; his breath a sigh, and his stooped hunch suggested a lifetime of poring over the lifelines of the rich and entitled.

Why and how he appeared on our doorstep, I have no idea. We weren't his usual clients. For a start we had no money, or that's what our father told us anyhow. And Dad wasn't about to part with the little he had to find out if his sons were going to America or if his daughters were marrying rich men next year, which appeared to be what the astrologer promised. I knew this because Sujata's parents, unlike ours, had money. They had been told that Sujata would marry a rich boy with an MBA from Harvard and have several boy children before she was thirty. Sujata's parents placed a large sum of money into the astrologer's open hands and praised his talents to all who cared to listen.

Maybe that's why he was at our place. From the outside, we looked entitled. We had a large home, a couple of servants, a garden where we grew sugarcane and we went to private schools. But Dad said we were living on borrowed money. Borrowed from uncles and grandfathers and cousins who lived in Africa. The sugarcane was supposed to make us enough money to pay back the rich cousins in Africa. Mum said it was another of Dad's grandiose schemes. It would come to nothing and we would all be tossed on the street when the cousins returned.

The astrologer disagreed. He knew he could change our fortunes. He sat cross-legged on the floor, resting his head briefly against the wall behind him. He drew lines across constellations and explained the power of the stars over our puny lives. His fingers were blue and yellow and his palms wrinkled and brown. Occasionally he looked hunted and we felt sorry for him, squinting at dusty books and charts and reading the futures of an ever-increasing number of people.

We stared, us kids, our mouths open at first then giggling behind our hands. Mum warned us with her eyes as he told us about Aquarius and Saturn and the moons in Venus and how we could, if we were clever, channel the power of those heavenly bodies before they harmed us. Because harm us, they would. Unless we diverted the wrath of the planetary gods away from us by choosing the right gemstones. Sapphire, diamond, cats-eye, topaz, ruby. He knew a gemstone dealer who could help. We must allow him to help us. Mum asked where the money for diamonds would come from. He ignored her and focussed his fierce eyes on Dad. He could see fortune, he told Dad; a home filled with happy, singing children, more money than we needed and certainly more than enough to place on his upturned palm after what he'd just told us. Mum said all that would be placed on his palm was a cup of tea. Dad laughed and said he could come back when everything he'd predicted came true.

The astrologer looked unhappy but bowed his head. When he coughed the air filled with rustling and thunder, and as he walked out we thought we saw planets revolving in the space above his head.

He came back, day after day, sitting stooped and cross-legged in the same position for hours, drawing, writing, sketching, and occasionally asking us questions. He seemed not to like us much. Occasionally I saw him frown terribly and mutter to himself. Intricate charts, however, emerged – Dad and the boys first of course. Dad's fortunes were espe- cially luminous; all the planets had kindly aligned at the hour of his birth to ensure an extremely long and prosperous life. He didn't need the enhancement of jewels. Sustained, regular donations of money to charity were recommended instead. Mum said homeless astrologers were considered charity cases, and wasn't that a nice coincidence.

Our brothers and cousins were next. Saturn and Pluto and Jupiter were explained over several cups of tea and samosas. Jewels were discussed. Topaz, amber, cats-eye, perhaps a yellow diamond for one of my brothers. To be worn on the index finger of the left hand. The oldest cousin could wear a diamond but sapphires were not recommended. Apart from Dad, it appeared all of us were in need of shiny interven- tions. Jewels that would augment the pathetic lives we were destined to lead because Saturn was in the ninth house and Mercury was rising and Jupiter ascending.

When he started doing my chart, it was on Mum's insistence. 'Why can't the girls also have their fortune told,' she said crossly. 'It's not like they aren't people too.' The astrologer resisted, trying to explain how my chart, like my stick-legged body, was still developing. Mum looked at him and he huffed and shuffled and said he would do his best.

He frowned as he wrote down the exact time of my birth, muttered and coughed as he calculated, shook his head to clear a blockage and finally stood up and walked out of the house. I had been watching him all day and ran to Mum and told her I was going to die. die.'

'Don't be so silly' she said.

'What else does it mean?' I wept. 'He was doing my chart. I will

'Oh yes, you're going to die,' my sister said. 'Because if you don't stop blubbering, I'll kill you.'

'Stop this nonsense, both of you.'

He came back a week later and summoned the family to his side.

My sister put her arm around me and looked worried.

'I have bad news,' the astrologer said. 'But it could be worse. It could have been one of the boys. However, it is the girl.'

'How dare you,' Mum said, pulling me away from my sister and putting her own arm around my shoulders. 'I've had enough of your rubbish. You are no longer welcome in this house.'

The astrologer looked at Dad. 'The girl is a mangli. Tuesday born. Under the influence of Saturn. No one can outrun a plane- tary influence like that. But here's the curious thing. I see a long life- line. So she will live. However, she must never marry. She will, umm, bring bad luck to the husband. Possibly death. I'm sorry. She's your responsibility for life, because if you give her to another family, you will be cursed. However, a sapphire will help ease that burden. Yes. You must get a sapphire ring at once.'

'Is that all?' I grinned and hugged Mum. 'I wasn't ever going to marry, anyway. Boys are so silly. Sister Mary Ascension says they are full of sin.'

'You're such a freak,' my sister pulled my hair and tapped my head before linking arms with me and dragging me out of the quiet room.

Our parents and brothers became more remote and less willing to mediate the fights I had with my sister when we were finally teenag- ers together. She fell in love with a sinful boy and married him and Mum watched me carefully for signs I might want to do the same one day.

'It's fine, Mum, don't worry,' I said to her at least once a day until she died. 'I have no desire to be a husband killer.'

And in my thirtieth year, as we watched the sun set over the Indian Ocean from the balcony of my house in Perth, my sister said casually, 'he killed himself, you know.'

'Who?'

'The astrologer who told you you'd be a spinster all your life that's who.'

'What?'

'Yes, shot himself. Very messy. One of the cousins found out about it and told mum.' My sister spoke slowly, her eyes distant, cup of tea forgotten.

'Why?'

'Nowadays we would recognise it as depression. Remember the signs? Didn't want to be around people, for a man whose profession put him in direct contact with people '

'How long have you known? And why have you waited 'til now to tell me this?'

'Mum told me before she died. Besides, none of the other stuff he said came true, anyway. Except for you.' She reached out and tapped the sapphire ring on my left hand as we thought about moons in Jupiter and suns in Saturn and the unfortunately short lives of both my husbands.

The right call?

Peter Rodgers

I'd prepared carefully for the talk with my dog, Asteroid, knowing it would be a turning point in our relationship. If I'd seen where it would lead, I'd have kept my mouth shut.

The talk was about life's hardest truth – that time runs out for us all. In Asteroid's case I'd decided it was more a question of money. I simply couldn't afford his vet bills anymore.

'I have some good news, and I have some bad news,' I told him. 'The good news is that I'm more than happy to go on feeding and housing you to the current high standard. There aren't many other dogs,' I added a bit smugly, 'who eat kangaroo fillet every second night. The bad news is that I've capped your future veterinary expenses at $1750. Once that's gone, so are you. In fact, the last $75 is earmarked for your final injection.'

Asteroid gave me one of his you must feel guilty to your core looks.

I broke the awkward silence saying, 'Of course, you can build up credit'.

'Just how can I do that?' he grumped, 'after all I'm only a dog.' 'Well, for a start, the rabbits are a problem in the garden. So for

each one you catch and show me there'll be a bonus of $30.' 'Why don't I just eat it?'

'Well, of course, and that would certainly save on kangaroo fillet, but I'll have to register it first.'

'Register it?'

'I bought this pocket ledger when I was at the newsagent earlier in the week.' I fished the smart red book out of my pocket and opened it to the first page. 'See, there's $1750 in your credit column already and nothing on the debit side. I think a $30 bonus per rabbit is entirely reasonable.'

'You've really worked it all out haven't you,' Asteroid said. His tone would have surprised those of my friends who were always going on about his angelic nature. 'And you know I have a problem with arthritis,' he added. 'I do, and that's why I'm more than happy to spend up on your krill oil tablets. But a bit more exercise would do you the world of good.'

Asteroid thought for a moment then said, 'Make it $40 a rabbit and I'll give it a go'.

'$35 tops, it's all I can afford.' 'Let's do it this way: $35 for the first six months, then $40.' 'You drive a hard bargain,' I said, with a relieved smile.

'Well, it's my life we're talking about here,' Asteroid replied. 'And if we're working out bonuses we're not going to stop at rabbits. What about all those visits to your mother? You know it gives her a lot of pleasure seeing me. That must count for something.'

'Fair point,' I agreed. 'For each future visit I'll add another $25.' 'Only $25!? Are you really saying that a dead rabbit is worth more

than your live Mum?'

'Of course not! But are you saying it's harder work visiting my mother than it is catching a rabbit? Don't push your luck.'

'Okay,' Asteroid conceded, 'but there are two other things; the first is that I can talk, the second is that I don't chase cats. Both of those have got to be worth serious dollars.'

'But all dogs, at least the ones I've had anything to do with, can communicate with their masters. It's—'.

'Communicate! What do you mean communicate?' Asteroid demanded, 'you and I talk. There's a world of difference and you know it. Think of all the conversations we've had over the years on everything from growing lettuces to Sophoclean tragedies to Sinus-American rivalry. When your wife ran away with the travel agent you told me it was only our heart-to-heart chats that got you through. I suppose you've forgotten all that!?'

'No, I haven't, and you have been a very special friend with very special talents and it's only right you've raised them now. I'll think about a bonus. By-the-way, it's Sino-American rivalry.'

'Is that so? Well, by-the-way,' he mimicked, 'please explain this nonsense about dogs and their masters. I've always regarded you as an equal.'

'Just a figure of speech,' I replied, 'don't take it to heart.' 'Cats?' Asteroid persisted.

'What about them?' I asked. 'Some dogs dislike them, others don't.

You just happen to be in the second category.'

'Sometimes you amaze me,' Asteroid said, shaking his head. 'I happen to be in the so-called second category only because of what you did to me as a pup. Yeah, I know you don't like to talk about it and I really do appreciate you calling me "him" in front of our friends. But rarely a day goes by when I don't wonder what it would be like to scare the living daylights out of a cat. I see one and my breathing gets shallow and my pulse quickens. A bit like you when you bring one of your girlfriends home and you're walking behind her to the house, I can practically see what you're thinking.' 'Excuse me!' I interrupted.

'I'm not trying to make you feel guilty, just the point that I may not act on my impulses the way other dogs do but I still feel some- thing, operation or no operation. I have to exercise self-control the way an alcoholic does.'

'I hardly think it's on a par with AA,' I said.

We sat in silence on the porch, looking out over the valley and the little puddles of smoke from early autumn fires. Asteroid gave me one of his serious looks and said, 'You do think that dogs are men's and women's best friend, don't you?'

'Of course I do,' I replied, 'without a doubt.'

'Don't you think it a bit odd that you've just put me on quota but you won't do the same for your Mum?'

'What on earth does she have to do with this?'

'Look at me. Overall, I'm in pretty reasonable shape, still enjoying life. Look at your Mum. Wonderful lady, I know, but there's only one way she'll leave the nursing home. Yet you go on pouring money into looking after her, strikes me as all a bit sad, not just for her but for you.'

'Now look here—,' I began. Asteroid cut me off.

'I know this is hard to hear, but if the ledger system is good enough for me, your best friend, it should be good enough for your other loved ones.'

'Just what are you getting at?' I asked.

'That we devise a rating system for humans and animals over a certain age,' he replied calmly. 'It would measure their quality of life and prospects and put a limit on how much would be spent on them.' 'Sounds suspiciously like euthanasia. And by animals I presume you mean dogs?'

'Well it's not really euthanasia, just that everyone would know exactly how much they have to play with, so to speak, and of course they'd be able to top it up by making themselves useful. You've provided the model in what you're doing with me. I'm simply suggesting we apply it more broadly. And yes, I do mean dogs, at least for a start. After all we're the ones closest to humans.'

'I thought monkeys had that honour, if that's the right word.' 'C'mon,' Asteroid despaired, 'monkeys might claim that but no

one in their right mind believes them. Just how many people keep monkeys as pets? When did you last see a sniffer monkey, let alone a guide one? Monkeys are out for themselves, end of story. Actually, I suppose that makes them very much like people. So okay then,' he shrugged, 'if you'd rather work with a monkey, fine by me, just give me the $1750 up front and I'll get out of your hair.'

'Alright, alright,' I said, 'calm down. Of course, I see us as a team. I just feel a bit nervous about what we're taking on.'

Our proposed rating system prompted parliamentary and pub debates across the nation, and a storm on social media. Many lauded our imagination and courage. We were given a 15-minute slot each week on ABC television called Earning Your Keep. It drew record audi- ences. Asteroid received approaches from major publishers for a prac- tical guide on teaching dogs to talk. He declined, saying they either had it them or they didn't. I felt that was a bit brusque, Asteroid insisted we concentrate on the job at hand.

We had our critics, especially in the media and the churches. 'Keep your paws off our Grannies!' screamed some the headlines. Prominent religious figures came out of, sometimes forced, retirement to lead a campaign against what they labelled, 'This evil book of death'. Our friends fretted about our well-being, but we laughed off their concerns. The vitriol was no worse than we'd expected. We persisted.

Then, that fateful Saturday when we travelled to Sydney to partic- ipate in a public debate at no less a venue than the Town Hall. It was a calm, sparkling evening, we arrived as the sun was setting behind the magnificent old building. It was great to be alive, to be pursuing a just and timely cause. We stood on the kerb opposite the Town Hall waiting for the lights to change. Suddenly, out of the crowd on the other side, a large, orange tabby cat appeared. It gave us a mean, challenging look.

Without warning, inexplicably, Asteroid took off, barrelling across the road. I yelled to him. He had eyes only for the cat. Asteroid was smart, incredibly smart. But he was no longer agile. He was also a country dog, unused to city traffic.

'These things do happen,' said the vet in the Haymarket, to where I rushed Asteroid in the back of a taxi after agreeing to pay triple fare to compensate for any blood stains. I cradled Asteroid all the way, he was comatose, I was in shock. The vet's tone was flat, nasal and completely uninterested. The closest he got to sympathy was another throw-away remark, 'If it makes you feel any better, he wouldn't have suffered much'. That did not help one jot. In the lonely days afterwards the only thing that salved my despair was the way Asteroid's many admirers rallied to keep his memory alive. Their efforts warmed and saddened me at the same time. Three months after his death, with the blessing of the Sydney City Council, we unveiled a small bronze plaque on the pavement opposite the Town Hall. It was nothing pretentious. But his lovingly sculpted image and the simple tribute, 'Asteroid – a true pioneer', reminded all who saw it of what we'd lost. A group of us shared the cost of the plaque. That worked out at exactly $75 each, the sum I'd allocated for Asteroid's farewell injection.

The irony of that figure still haunts me. Much worse, I've betrayed the cause for which Asteroid died. In my defence, I could point to the fact that the police urged me to adopt a low profile, as they put it, and my friends tell me I'm just being prudent. But I feel a profound sense of shame. The terrible truth is that I lack the courage of my convictions.

The day after the memorial ceremony I received a voicemail from someone claiming to represent The Friends of Life. The message said: 'We got the dog, we'll get you if we have to, and we won't use a cat. Your call.'

I had no choice really. Did I?

Water the Colour of Clay

Hollen Pockets

There is significant rainfall. Astrid knows this for certain because she has a pluviometer. She notes the millimetres of rain like some watch the stock market. The reading rises and falls. No one ever says anything definitive about its meaning. She tells people about her measurements, compares them with the Bureau of Meteorology readings. Rainfall isn't something that people like to talk to her about but she had predicted the January season. Every day, the last four days, it has bucketed down. In between torrents, her garden gasps for sunlight and tries to absorb the puddles. Astrid watches it now, her hydrangeas trying to lift their blue bobbles to make eye-contact with the sun.

'Do you want to go for a swim?'

The gutters are filling up. The storm drains are as old as their house. Astrid has called the council about them before, twice, but nothing has ever been done. Today, she will not call. They have enough on their plate.

'Swim?'

The sky turned bottle-green the day Beau was born. Hail fell and Astrid's water broke. They had to drive to hospital in the storm. Pebbles of ice pelted the station wagon the whole way there. Nav drove slowly, afraid of aquaplaning. Astrid watched ice bouncing off the windscreen. The sky is falling and the baby is coming.

'The largest hailstone ever recorded fell on . . . Vivian, South Dakota!' Astrid yelped between arcs of pain. 'It weighed in at almost .

. . one kilo with a fifty . . . fifty centimetre circumference.' She breathed and breathed ss-ss-ss breaths.

'I can't drive faster. We'll get there.' Nav was almost shouting over the din. 'I love you, just as an aside. It's not important to say it right now because we're not in any kind of trouble. I'm a fantastic driver, ask anyone.'

'It's almost impossible to calculate the terminal . . . velocity of a hailstone,' Astrid replied. 'There are so many factors.'

Beau came early for no reason and weighed only a little more than the recordbreaking, South Dakota hailstone. He came out small and round, almost fitting in the palm of Nav's hand.

'Come on.' Nav fans his eyelashes.

'The pool is closed. It's a disaster out there, don't you know? The meteorology forums are going absolutely bananas.'

Nav loves to swim in the rain. The hot weather fuels him. He glows in the summer. When the weather congests into roiling humidity, Nav basks. When the hot streak breaks, in that Australian way, straight into torrential rain, that is his favourite time to swim. He always jumps in first.

'The rain makes the pool water warmer.'

Astrid believed him, or rather, she didn't think too hard about it. She preferred to live in his tangible belief, to splash around in the tepid pool water under the cold, falling sheets and think, as he does, that the feeling is causal and not just contrast.

Later that evening, they gird themselves to go next door to collect their son. Beau has spent the day there with Sofie Giordano. She is twelve, two years older than Beau but she seems to like playing with him. Everyone likes Beau.

It had taken them eight years of living next to each other to do more than nod hello to their fancier neighbours. Beau bridged the divide when they got him a trampoline. The Giordanos also have a trampoline. The children from opposite sides of the fence had become friends, eight feet in the air. Beau, despite being the youngest, is an excellent bouncer.

Nav and Astrid dash over to the neighbour's house with coats pulled over their heads. Sofie's mother, Evaline Giordano greets them with a smile that powers up her face, a dimmer light bulb on its way to maximum brightness. They follow her skirt-hem up the stairs. On the landing, they pass a wheeled suitcase.

'Precious memories,' Evaline points to it. 'Photo albums, baby hair, everything. I put it here in case the lower level floods.'

Astrid actually knows how high the Hunter floods of the 1950s reached—some of the older houses in town have tidelines—but she keeps this information to herself.

They find Sofie is thrashing Beau on the Nintendo. 'I'm staying over,' Beau signs to his parents. 'Sofie says.'

Astrid suspects that a lot of parents would like Beau a lot less if they could read Auslan.

'Ask nicely,' Nav signs.

Beau pulls his phone out and starts texting: Please may I stay? Sofie was going to show me her ant-farm and then her telescope later if the rain stops. Beau presses the phone into Evaline's hands and stands waiting, expressive eyes, luminous with hope. He signs the word for please, spelling it out letter by letter instead of as a single word and slow enough that Sofie's mother can follow. Evaline Giordano doesn't stand a chance.

Tipper is waiting for them at the door and, upon their much-antic- ipated return, does frenzied laps of the living room – up and down the furniture.

Tipper is a kelpie-cross, intelligent and easy to train but highly energetic. These are the facts Astrid learned about the breed after Nav brought the little thing home. They're meant to be working dogs, roving alongside a farmer with a ute, hustling sheep and cattle, fighting snakes and digging holes.

'It's a runt,' Nav persuaded her. 'It needs us.'

After being in the enormous, well-insulated Giordano place, their home feels flimsy and the sound of the rain is amplified. Their house is old, almost Federation, so the noise of rain on the tin roof rattles like a snare drum.

Astrid and Nav are parents left alone with each other in the rarefied, lockdown atmosphere of the storm. They are both damp and chilled. Astrid runs a shower and draws Nav in with her. It's not special, like swimming under an open sky, but the water is hot and the noise of the shower, of them, is underscored by the unrelenting rain.

Beau returns at midday the next day. The sun broke free that morning and is dancing for joy on every surface, pools and puddles and droplets. Nav is at work and Astrid is on the porch with Tipper curled under the cane chair. Astrid is half-working, skim reading articles she might want to actually read.

'Want to go to the river?' Beau signs to her the moment she looks up.

'Greetings, my only son! I see you have returned. I am well. How goes it with you?'

'Greetings, Mother,' Beau replies, sarcastically. 'May we please go to the river?'

It turns out the Hunter is making real threats to flood the town. Overnight, it spilled its banks and filled the football fields and parkland between the riverbed and the main street.

It takes Astrid, her son and the dog only ten minutes to walk from home to the new location of the river. Tipper prances around them the whole time they're walking. Almost from the day they got her, she hasn't needed a lead. She sticks to their ankles and stops at roads to cross with them. Intelligent, easy to train, highly energetic.

The embankment, below which are usually soccer pitches and playgrounds and trails, is busy with people taking photos, walking their own dogs, marvelling at the change. The river has expanded to a fat, pulsing torrent that ends right at the lip of the embankment. If the waters were to rise even ten centimetres, it will overtop the embank- ment and start on the shops and houses. The water is brown and foamy and full of detritus – tree branches and garbage and, most strangely, the occasional watermelon. These green orbs race by, new ones appear- ing at steady intervals, bobbing and weaving in the rapid waters.

They walk along the embankment, following the river. It surges quickest at the centre and the waters at the edge are almost still, swirling slower. It is impeded there by benches, sheds and the tops of trees emerging from the muddy stew, jacarandas, willows and euca- lypts.

They pass lots of people making the same walk, strangers and some people they know from town. They all smile at each other and sometimes stop to speak, exchange adjectives for the mess of the river and speculate about the fate of their town. There's a festive feeling in the air, like when you meet people out looking at Christmas lights or at a parade. No one looks worried, everyone seems excited. They pass the bridge, lined with people. As the best vantage point, it makes for a natural gathering point. Beyond that point, the walk is less populous. Eventually, they reach a non-submerged bench and Astrid sits. It's an interesting view. Here, the river has flooded natural parkland and is forced to weave through dense treetops. One eucalypt has fallen, leaning out over the river on a canopy of other, still-standing trees.

'We'll go back in a minute, go up and take a look from the bridge on the way home?'

Beau nods, sitting next to her feet on the damp ground, pulling up wads of grass. Astrid shuts her eyes, enjoying the spangled sunlight reflecting off the river. After a minute, Beau puts a hand on her arm.

'Can I go climb on the fallen-down tree?' 'No, of course not. That's super dangerous.' 'Tipper's doing it, she's fine.'

Astrid stands, heart thudding. The dog, still a puppy really, is skipping along the eucalypt's body, darting around branches and sniffing all along.

'Oh, god!' Astrid whistles. Kelpies are intelligent, easy to train, and Tipper's head whips around. She clambers over a spray of leaves and

locks eyes with Astrid. It occurs to Astrid that whistling may have been a mistake as the kelpie pup, rather than taking the long way back along the tree trunk, leaps into the clay-coloured slurry and vanishes.

'Shit!' Astrid immediately sees a vision of Nav's devastated face in her mind. Beau laughs, not yet reading her concern. Dogs can swim, everyone knows that, and with a child's optimism, Beau doesn't realise the diving dog might not come back up. Astrid can't see her.

The river is opaque even one centimetre down from the surface, more dirt soup than water. She runs along the foamy lip of the flood, whistling and calling for the underwater dog. Beau shadows Astrid, beginning to catch her fear.

She kneels on the tree and stretches herself out, dunking her arms in the water, feeling around for the submerged dog. Astrid knows this is daft. She isn't even far enough out on the gum, the silly pup hopped in from much further along. It's too dangerous, she can't follow the kelpie out there on this wrecked tree. She also can't stop scooping her arms through the water because, when she does, she will have to tell Beau what she already knows. Then later, she'll have to tell Nav. He will understand and Beau will not. She has lost the dog. She called it and it jumped, of course it did. Tears are forming behind her eyes and she scratches her hand on god-knows-what, something that is both slimy and sharp, and she's muddy and the dog is gone and it was only a runt.

Beau stands on her foot, pressing down deliberately to get her attention. He's soaked to the stomach and holding a drenched Tipper, wriggling happily in his arms.

Astrid grabs her filthy son by the shoulders.

'You didn't get in for the damn dog?' Astrid knows the answer.

Beau shakes his head and slips, muddily, out of her grasp, his tell-tale sneakers squelching and squeaking.

Tipper drops out of Beau's arms and shakes, misting both her owners with an extra smattering of river-water. Somewhere, while swimming, the kelpie found a tennis ball, heavy and ancient. She coughs it up at her owner's feet and sits, making meaningful eye-contact with her favourite person, quivering with energy but well-trained.

www.ingramcontent.com/pod-product-compliance
Lightning Source LLC
Chambersburg PA
CBHW021702110726

47902CB00007B/2034
9780995440913